Gamut Index of Skeletal Dysplasias

D1522929

Springer

London
Berlin
Heidelberg
New York
Barcelona
Hong Kong
Milan
Paris
Singapore
Tokyo

Kazimierz Kozlowski and Peter Beighton

Gamut Index of Skeletal Dysplasias

An Aid to Radiodiagnosis

Third Edition

Foreword by John Masel

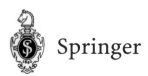 Springer

Kazimierz Kozlowski, MRACR, Doc
Honorary Radiologist, Royal Alexandra Hospital for Children, Sydney, Australia

Peter Beighton, MD, PhD, FRCP, FRCPCH, FRSSA
Emeritus Professor of Human Genetics, University of Cape Town Medical School,
Observatory 7925, Cape Town, South Africa

ISBN 1-85233-365-0 Springer-Verlag London Berlin Heidelberg

British Library Cataloguing in Publication Data
Kozlowski, Kazimierz, 1928–
    Gamut index of skeletal dysplasias: an aid to radiodiagnosis. – 3rd ed.
    1. Human skeleton – Abnormalities – Diagnosis
    2. Human skeleton – Radiography   3. Diagnosis, Radioscopic
    I. Title   II. Beighton, Peter
    616.7'1'043
    ISBN 1852333650

Library of Congress Cataloging-in-Publication Data
Gamut index of skeletal dysplasias: an aid to radiodiagnosis/Kazimierz Kozlowski and Peter Beighton;
    foreword by John Masel. – 3rd ed.
        p. cm.
    Includes index.
    ISBN 1-85233-365-0 (alk. paper)
    1. Human skeleton – Abnormalities – Diagnosis. 2. Diagnosis, Radioscopic I. Beighton, Peter. II. Title
    RD761.K69 2001
    616.7'1043–dc21   00-063760

Typeset by Gray Publishing, Tunbridge Wells, Kent, England
Printed and bound by Athenæum Press, Gateshead, Tyne and Wear, England
28/3830-543210 Printed on acid-free paper SPIN 10778388

To our good friend and colleague

Bryan Cremin

in recognition of his achievements in paediatric radiology
and for his unfailing good humour and generosity of spirit.

Foreword

The publication of a third edition after only five years confirms the widespread popularity of this book.

Apart from the numerous additions and modifications consequent on the substantial expansion of knowledge in this field, the authors have further improved the value of this text with the excellent chapter, as mentioned in their preface, on general aspects of the problem. The advances referred to in this chapter, particularly molecular genetics and database access, have transformed the diagnosis of skeletal dysplasias. However, this basic text remains an essential starting point for anyone confronted with an unfamiliar condition.

Among the references listed on page xix, Dr Kozlowski's paper 'The radiographic clues in the diagnosis of bone dysplasias', Pediatric Radiology 1985; 15: 1–3, is still essential reading.

John Masel

Preface to the First Edition

The skeleton is involved to a significant extent in more than 500 genetic and congenital syndromes and although the majority of these are individually rare, collectively they are not uncommon. Diagnostic precision, which is crucial for accurate prognostication and effective management, is frequently dependent upon recognition of radiological stigmata. For this reason the radiologist plays a key role in the appraisal and investigation of persons with disorders of this type. With these points in mind we have written this handbook for use in the radiographic reporting room. We have endeavored to provide the essential information which will facilitate radiodiagnosis and have striven for clarity and accuracy. We believe that our objective will be achieved by means of the "gamut" format which we have employed.

In Section 1 we have addressed the problem of diagnosis of generalised skeletal abnormalities, while Section 2 is based upon an anatomical or regional approach. Lists of conditions are given in order of prevalence or importance. Our gamut has been deliberately simplified and only the most important and easily recognised radiographic stigmata have been taken into account. Pertinent clinical, radiographic, and genetic information for each syndromic entity is provided in Section 3, where the disorders are placed in alphabetical order. This section also contains relevant references which are as up to date as possible. The majority relate to clinical and radiographic reviews which will be of practical value. After due consideration we have restricted these, with few exceptions, to the English language as these will be most readily available to the majority of readers. We have also appended references to general review articles and monographs which have direct relevance to the radiodiagnosis of genetic and congenital skeletal syndromes.

As far as possible we have employed the terminology of the 1983 version of the provisional Paris Nomenclature, which is set out in Appendix B. In line with current practice, the possessive forms of eponyms have been avoided, but names or descriptive designations which are in everyday usage have been retained.

As with many aspects of life, it is often difficult to know where to stop, and we have made arbitrary decisions concerning the inclusion or exclusion of many disorders. In general we have tried to mention every well-established entity while excluding "private syndromes" which have been reported only in a single individual or kindred. For the sake of differential diagnosis and completion, clinically important nongenetic disorders appear at the end of each gamut list. However, as our book is primarily concerned with inherited skeletal dysplasia syndromes we have made no attempt to provide any details of these acquired conditions. For this information the reader is referred to the standard textbooks of radiology, where they are fully described and discussed.

The majority of the genetic disorders of bone are most easily diagnosed in childhood, and in later life the radiographic appearances may be nonspecific. For these reasons our gamut lists primarily concern the first and second decades and disorders of adulthood have been omitted.

This book is based upon knowledge and experience acquired in Europe, America, South Africa, and the Antipodes; it was conceived in Sydney and parturition took place in Cape Town. We trust that the heterogeneity of its origins will enhance its value to colleagues throughout the world.

Sydney and Cape Town
1983

Kazimierz Kozlowski
Peter Beighton

Preface to Second Edition

The first edition of the Gamut Index was published a decade ago. Since that time, many new skeletal disorders have been delineated and we have prepared this second edition in order to encompass this additional material. The Gamut has been written for general and paediatric radiologists but it will also be of interest to paediatricians and orthopaedic surgeons, as well as trainees and residents in these specialities.

The format, as described in the Preface to the first edition, is essentially unchanged although the gamut lists in section 1 and 2 have been supplemented and expanded. In section 3, brief descriptions of additional skeletal conditions have been added and in order to facilitate access to further information, numerical designations from McKusick's Catalogue of Inherited Disorders, "Mendelian Inheritance in Man" (MIM) have been appended to the titles of these disorders in Section 3.

The list of relevant Textbooks and Monographs in Appendix A has been revised and in Appendix B the "Paris Nomenclature 1983" has been replaced by the "International Classification of Osteochondrodysplasias 1992". We have included every disorder that appears in the Classification, together with others culled from the literature, but for sake of clarity and simplicity, excessive rarities and private syndromes have been purposely omitted. In the same way, references have been chosen in order to provide up to date information which is relevant to radiodiagnosis.

We have received many positive comments concerning the value of the first edition and we hope that this new version will prove to be equally useful to our colleagues and friends.

Sydney and Cape Town
1994

Kazimierz Kozlowski
Peter Beighton

Preface to the Third Edition

Diagnostic precision is essential for effective management and meaningful medical and genetic prognostication. In the skeletal dysplasias, diagnosis is based to a large extent upon the recognition of characteristic radiographical features. The first edition of the Gamut Index was published in 1984 and the second in 1995. New skeletal dysplasias continue to be documented, while existing conditions are proving to be increasingly heterogeneous, hence the need for this new edition.

We have now included a chapter embracing concepts that relate to the diagnosis of the skeletal dysplasias. These include the significance of syndromic associations, antenatal diagnosis by imaging techniques, aspects of laboratory diagnosis and the role of electronic databases.

It must be emphasised that the field of bone dysplasias is becoming increasingly complex. This gamut is intended for the general radiologist and experts who require detailed information are referred to the standard textbooks that are listed in Appendix A. Equally, although all conditions which are listed in the 1997 International Classification and Nomenclature of the Osteochondrodysplasias are mentioned in Section III and appear in the Gamut lists, we have excluded disorders which are excessively rare. In order to clarify the increasingly confusing nosology, identification numbers that appear in successive editions of McKusick's Catalogue of Mendelian Disorders in Man (MIM) are quoted and cross-referenced in the Gamut. The molecular basis of the individual skeletal dysplasias is rapidly being elucidated and future re-classification on a basis of the underlying defects of the genes and gene products can be foreseen.

The references concerning the specific conditions in Section III have been revised and updated. Wherever possible these pertain to reviews or articles that are of relevance in radiological practice. It is significant, however, that the era of descriptive syndromic delineation is now over, and that the majority of contemporary articles concerning the skeletal dysplasias are focussed upon molecular advances. For the sake of brevity, references to publications concerning molecular defects have generally been omitted. Those that have been included contain reviews or bibliographies that are pertinent to radiodiagnosis.

Both authors have now reached the age of 65 years, and consequently experienced mandatory retirement. We wish to place on record the academic satisfaction that we have derived from writing successive editions of the Gamut and the harmony in which we have worked together.

Sydney and Cape Town
2000

Kazimierz Kozlowski
Peter Beighton

Diagnosis of the Bone Dysplasias

1. Syndromic Associations

There are only a few bone dysplasias in which the manifestations are restricted to the skeletal system. In the majority other body systems are also involved, in the form of associated abnormalities or secondary complications. For these reasons there are no clear-cut distinctions between bone dysplasias and "syndromic associations." In general, however, multiple congenital anomaly syndromes and multiple anomalies/mental retardation syndromes show less severe and less characteristic bony features. These bone changes are polyostotic (not generalised) and the pattern of skeletal involvement is variable in location and severity.

Many common bone dysplasias are associated with dermatological conditions including disorders of epidermis, dermis, sebaceous glands, hair and nails. Altered pigmentation, tumour and tumourous-like abnormalities may also be involved. Knowledge of these associations is important, as diagnosis may be problematical in some bone dysplasias unless the specific skin changes are also present. For instance, recognition of neurofibromatosis and McCune-Albright syndrome is difficult unless the characteristic cutaneous pigmentary changes are recognised. Similarly, malformed or absent nails are a constant finding in the nail-patella syndrome, while a diagnosis of the McKusick form of metaphyseal dysplasia is unlikely in patients with normal hair.

Immunological defects in bone dysplasias may involve B cells, T cells, phagocytosis or complement systems. The most common of these disorders is the Schwachman syndrome. Further examples of bone dysplasia-immunodeficiency syndromes are immunodeficiency-short limb dwarfism and the hyper IGE syndrome with osteopenia. Haematological abnormalities are uncommon but distinctive features of some bone dysplasias, such as Schwachman syndrome, some osteosclerotic bone dysplasias and diaphyseal dysplasia with anaemia.

Heart and kidney abnormalities are common in the "neonatal death dwarfism" group of bone dysplasias but are rare in children who survive the first few years of life. There are few exceptions, however, such as chondroectodermal dysplasia and Schimke immuno-osseous dysplasia.

Neurologic abnormalities in the bone dysplasias may be primary or secondary. Primary severe malformations of the central nervous system are common in bone dysplasias that have an early fatal outcome. Secondary neurological complications are consequent upon the underlying primary bone abnormalities. The most common and most important of these are cranio-cervical junction malformations (small foramen magnum, subluxation/dislocation C1/C2) which result in cranio-cervical compression. Other well known neurological complications are those which follow progressive kyphosis and scoliosis. In patients with cervical kyphosis (diastrophic dysplasia, campomelic dysplasia) neurological dysfunction may appear early in life. Spinal stenosis rarely causes complications in childhood. In the sclerosing bone dysplasias, osseous overgrowth and foraminal obstruction leads to cranial nerve compression. Mental retardation is rare in patients with bone dysplasias who survive the first few years of life. Minor or uncharacteristic bone changes in persons with mental retardation are a feature of chromosomal abnormalities and mental retardation/bone dysplasia syndromes. Dysharmonic maturation in the bone dysplasias may result from increased or decreased blood flow due to any cause.

2. Radiological Diagnosis of Bone Dysplasias

Many bone dysplasias are recognised only late in life especially if the clinical history is inadequate or vital clinical signs are overlooked. The following "hints" from the case history and clinical findings would suggest the diagnosis of a bone dysplasia or syndromic association:

i.	History of a similar disorder in the family.
ii.	Family members with short stature.
iii.	Joint contractures or joint laxity.
iv.	Unusual gait.
v.	Hands and/or feet deformities.
vi.	Abnormalities of other tissues/organs (e.g. unusual face, abnormal nose, eyes, ears, dermatological or neurological abnormalities).

For radiographic diagnosis, seven basic views are necessary:

i.	Lateral skull.
ii.	Lateral spine.
iii.	Pelvis and hips with lower lumbar spine (AP).
iv.	Chest including shoulders (PA).
v.	Legs including knees and ankles.
vi.	Arms including elbows.
vii.	Hands and wrists

If all seven radiographs are normal, a bone dysplasia can be excluded. If changes are present, but the diagnosis cannot be reached on the basis of these seven radiographs, then full skeletal survey is indicated. Radiographs are sometimes sent for a consultant opinion; it is essential that these films should be accompanied by pertinent clinical and biochemical data. Properly organised documents sent for consultation include:

i. Detailed clinical history.
ii. Photographs of the patient, including the whole body and face.
iii. Basic laboratory "bone screening tests" – serum calcium, phosphorus and alkaline phosphatase levels.
iv. Cytogenetic findings if the patient is mentally retarded.
v. CT and/or MR of the head in appropriate circumstances.

CT and/or MRI of the skull are indicated in all persons with Bone Dysplasia–Mental Retardation syndromes. In addition, for prognostication special radiographs/CT/MR may be necessary. For instance, of the neck if hypoplastic/dysplastic changes in the suboccipital region are suspected, or to demonstrate the spinal canal contents when malsegmentation, severe kyphosis or scoliosis of the spine are present.

3. Antenatal Diagnosis of Bone Dysplasias

Ultrasonic investigation of the unborn child has proved to be of great value in the bone dysplasias. Routine ultrasonic procedures, which are harmless and non-invasive, provide an efficient means of appraisal of the foetal skeleton. In particular, the dimensions, configuration and presence or absence of skeletal components can readily be determined. In this way, antenatal surveillance of a potentially "at risk" pregnancy can be undertaken. Information concerning the duration of pregnancy is an essential factor in this process.

Sonography in pregnancy has considerable relevance for the antenatal diagnosis of bone dysplasias as the discovery of skeletal abnormalities may be followed by a request for termination of pregnancy. Whereas the precise diagnosis by conventional radiography of lethal neonatal bone dysplasias and those appearing early in life is excellent, the specific ultrasound diagnosis of antenatal bone dysplasias is accurate in only about 50% of instances. As osteogenesis imperfecta is the most common bone dysplasia diagnosed at birth, it is also most frequently suspected on ultrasound examination.

Aborted foetuses are often presented for radiographic confirmation of the diagnosis; it is relevant that the difficulties in radiographic analysis and diagnosis are inversely proportional to the age of the foetus. The earlier the termination is performed, the more difficult it is to make a radiological diagnosis. For this reason, histological examination of cartilage is indicated in all undiagnosed or doubtful cases. In the future, molecular genetic testing may be the decisive final examination.

Diagnostic sonography should be performed only in centres that have special experience. In particular, without sonographic expertise, unnecessary pregnancy termination of normal foetuses or those with regressive long bone bowing may be performed.

4. Laboratory Diagnosis

In bone dysplasias with defective mineralisation (osteoporosis and osteosclerosis), basic biochemical tests often yield abnormal findings. For this reason, routine blood and urine examinations and estimations of serum levels of calcium, phosphorus and alkaline phosphatase are necessary in the investigation of conditions in these categories. Similarly, the dysostosis multiplex group of disorders usually requires investigation of mucopolysaccharides and complex carbohydrates for final diagnosis. Otherwise, with a few exceptions such as Wolcott–Rallison dysplasia and Kenny–Caffey dysplasia, biochemical screening tests are normal in the majority of genetic bone dysplasias.

Molecular genetics is playing an increasingly important role in the elucidation of the bone dysplasias. The chromosomal loci of the determinant genes have been defined in many of these conditions, facilitating pre-symptomatic and antenatal diagnosis by "gene tracking" techniques in appropriate families. In some bone dysplasias, the actual structure of the molecular abnormalities has been determined (gene characterisation) and in others the faulty gene product has been identified. It is of importance, however, that the molecular basis of many bone dysplasias is far from straight forward. For instance, disparate conditions may result from faults in the same gene, while clinically similar disorders may have different underlying molecular defects. Despite this complexity, there is little doubt that molecular investigations will have considerable diagnostic implications in the near future. For these reasons, an understanding of this rapidly developing field is necessary for all professionals who have an interest in the bone dysplasias.

5. Informatics

Information concerning genetic disorders, including the skeletal dysplasias is available on a number of electronic databases. The most widely used of these is the online version of McKusick's Catalogue of "Mendelian Inheritance in Man", (OMIM) which is constantly updated and accessible on **http://www.ncbi.nlm.nih.gov/omim.**

The Index Medicus, which is an important source of references, can be researched on Medline at **http://www.ncbi.nlm.nih.gov/Entrez/medline.html**. The diagnostic process is facilitated by interactive databases such as the London Dysmorphology Data Base (**http://genetics.ich.ucl.ac.uk/lddb/lddb.html**) and the Australian equivalent "POSSUM". The latter includes "OSSUM" which is devoted to skeletal dysplasias.

Conventional atlases of genetic bone disorders are listed in the Appendix; this format is also moving with the times and electronic versions are becoming available. The "Radiological Electronic Atlas of Malformation Syndromes and Skeletal Dysplasias" (REAMS) has already appeared and it is likely that others will follow. The Internet is a rich source of medical information, albeit often subjective, for those with the time to browse or the ability to fast track. Digitalisation of imagery and electronic transmission is yet another rapidly developing field, which has clear implications for radiological diagnosis of the skeletal dysplasias.

6. Museum Specimens

Although the diagnosis of skeletal dysplasias is largely dependent on radiographs, it is relevant that these films are two-dimensional representations of three-dimensional reality. Valuable insights can be obtained from the examination of the actual skeletons of persons with bone dysplasias, but these are few and far between. Nevertheless, extensive collections of skeletons of this type are to be found in the Museums of Pathological Anatomy, Vienna, and the Vrolik Collection, University of Amsterdam. Other specimens are exhibited in the museum of the Royal College of Surgeons, London, and the Institute of Pathological Anatomy, University of Munich.

References (Diagnosis)

Beighton P, Sujansky E, Patzak B, Portele KA (1993). Genetic skeletal dysplasias in the Museum of Pathological Anatomy, Vienna. Am J Med Genet 47:843–847

Beighton P, Sujansky E, Patzak B, Portele KA (1994). Bone dysplasias of infancy in the Vienna collection. Pediatr Radiol 24:284–286

Harlow CL, Kilcoyne RF, Aeling J, Becker MH (1997). Skin and bones: dermatologic conditions with skeletal abnormalities. Skeletal Radiol 26:201–213

Kozlowski K (1985). The radiographic clues in the diagnosis of bone dysplasias. Pediatr Radiol 15:1–3

Nerlich AG, Freisinger P (1998). Severe rhizomelic skeletal dysplasia in a museum skeleton. Skeletal Radiol 27:46–49

Oostra RJ, Baljet B, Dijkstra PF, Hennekam RCM (1998). Congenital anomalies in the teratological collection of the Museum Vrolik in Amsterdam, The Netherlands. II. Skeletal dysplasias. Am J Med Genet 77:116–134

Acknowledgements

We are grateful to many people who have been involved in the production of this book. We offer our special thanks to John P. Masel of Brisbane, for his painstaking scrutiny of the contents and for his constructive comments on all three editions. Greta Beighton prepared the manuscript and index with her customary enthusiasm, efficiency and good humour which she has retained throughout four decades of interaction and collaboration. Without her informatic skills and dedicated approach, it is most unlikely that the publishing deadlines would have been met.

This book has been based in part upon experience obtained during more than three decades of investigations supported by the Mauerberger Foundation, the South African Medical Research Council, and the University of Cape Town Staff Research Fund. PB acknowledges with gratitude support received from Chirosciences-Celltech during the preparation of the third edition of this book.

Contents

Introduction – How to Use This Book

If generalised radiological changes are present, choose the appropriate category on the first page of Section 1, and then consult the relevant gamut list. When abnormalities are confined to specific regions of the skeleton, Section 2 should be consulted in the same way.

The index contains the numbers of other pages where the condition in question also appears. By cross-reference, the reader should be in a position to make a provisional diagnosis. The diagnosis can be confirmed by consulting Section 3, where essential clinical, radiological and genetic information for each syndrome is summarised. These conditions are listed in alphabetical order and alternative designations are given. Key references are provided in case further information is required.

Appendix A contains a list of monographs concerning the skeletal dysplasia syndromes in which these disorders are depicted and described in detail. Finally, in order to resolve any terminological problems, the latest version of the International nomenclature is provided in Appendix B.

Section 1

Generalised Skeletal Abnormalities

1.1   Osteoporosis

Generalised osteoporosis that is recognised radiologically is usually indicative of severe metabolic dysfunction. Less often, widespread osteoporosis is encountered as a component of an inherited bone dysplasia. Multiple fractures and/or pseudofractures complicate many of these conditions.

1.1.1   Skeletal Dysplasias with Osteoporosis

Massive osteoporosis and a fracturing tendency are important signs of osteogenesis imperfecta and a few other rare bone dysplasias. These manifestations are most severe at birth and decrease with age in the forms of these conditions that are non-lethal. In terms of pathogenesis, a distinction can be drawn between osteoporosis and osteomalacia, but as the former term is in widespread use we have used it in this non-specific sense throughout this book.

1.1.1.1	Osteogenesis Imperfecta (heterogeneous)
1.1.1.2	Osteogenesis Imperfecta, variant forms (Bruck, Grant, Cole–Carpenter syndromes)
1.1.1.3	Juvenile Idiopathic Osteoporosis
1.1.1.4	Achondrogenesis

1.1.2   Inherited Metabolic Disorders with Osteoporosis

1.1.2.1	Hypophosphataemia (Vitamin D-resistant Rickets)
1.1.2.2	Other Genetic Forms of Metabolic and Renal Rickets with or without Secondary Hyperparathyroidism.
1.1.2.3	Hyperparathyroidism
1.1.2.4	Complex Carbohydrate Metabolic Disorders (Mucopolysaccharidoses, MPS, and Mucolipidoses, MLS)
1.1.2.5	Hypophosphatasia

1.1.3   Other Rare Genetic Disorders Manifesting Osteoporosis

1.1.3.1	Metaphyseal Chondrodysplasia, Jansen type
1.1.3.2	Focal Dermal Hypoplasia (Goltz Syndrome)

Generalised Skeletal Abnormalities

1.1.3.3	Cockayne Syndrome
1.1.3.4	Singleton–Merten Syndrome
1.1.3.5	Geroderma Osteodysplastica Hereditaria
1.1.3.6	Cerebro-oculo-facio-skeletal Syndrome
1.1.3.7	Parastremmatic Dysplasia
1.1.3.8	Transient Painful Osteoporosis of the Legs
1.1.3.9	Homocystinuria
1.1.3.10	Thalassaemia Major
1.1.3.11	Osteoectasia with Hyperphosphatasia
1.1.3.12	Idiopathic Hypercalciuria
1.1.3.13	Menkes Kinky Hair Syndrome
1.1.3.14	Glycogen Storage Disease
1.1.3.15	Osteoporosis-pseudoglioma Syndrome
1.1.3.16	Osteopenia with Radiolucent Lesions of the Mandible
1.1.3.17	HyperIGE Syndrome with Osteopenia
1.1.3.18	Cranioectodermal Dysplasia

1.1.4   Osteolyses, Idiopathic

The osteolyses present with radiographic lucency of the skeleton and they enter into the differential diagnosis of "osteoporosis". They are conventionally classified into the "acro-osteolyses" or "peripheral" forms (see 2.6.5) and the "generalised" or "multicentric forms". In practice, there is considerable overlap, and precise categorisation may be difficult. The multicentric forms, which are listed below, must be distinguished from the massive osteolysis of Gorham:

1.1.4.1	Winchester Syndrome
1.1.4.2	Torg Type of Generalised Osteolysis
1.1.4.3	Mandibulo-acral Dysplasia
1.1.4.4	Familial Expansile Osteolysis

1.1.5   Acquired or Non-genetic Osteoporosis

Osteoporosis is a major feature of many non-genetic disorders and non-specific chronic disease of many types (see 1.2.5). These conditions enter into the radiological differential diagnosis of the skeletal dysplasia syndromes, and for the sake of completion, they are listed below:

1.1.5.1	Non-genetic Metabolic, Renal, and Dietary Rickets
1.1.5.2	Prolonged Immobilisation
1.1.5.3	Leukaemia and Other Small Cell Tumours

1.2 Multiple Fractures

Multiple fractures are characteristic of a number of inherited bone dysplasias and metabolic disorders. Each of these conditions is usually accompanied by additional and often diagnostic radiographic features. Osteoporosis is usually but not invariably present. Osteogenesis imperfecta is more common than all the other fragile bone disorders put together. Idiopathic osteoporosis is differentiated by its occurrence in mid-childhood. Osteogenesis imperfecta should not be confused with battered child syndrome. The differential diagnosis is usually easy and a lateral skull radiograph (Wormian bones) is often helpful; in some instances nuclear scan may be of value. Fractures can be the first manifestation in osteoporotic bone disease, but they also occur in some osteosclerotic skeletal disorders, notably osteopetrosis and pycnodysostosis. Other causes of pathological fractures include neurological disorders, bone tumours and osteomyelitis. In rare instances, stress fractures can mimic bone dysplasias.

1.2.1 Skeletal Dysplasias with Predominant Bone Fragility

1.2.2   Metabolic Disorders with Fractures or Pseudofractures

Pseudofractures are a well-recognised feature of many forms of rickets. In extreme circumstances true fractures may also occur in these disorders (see 1.1.4).

1.2.2.1	Hypophosphataemic Rickets
1.2.2.2	Genetic Forms of Metabolic and Renal Rickets
1.2.2.3	Hypophosphatasia
1.2.2.4	Non-genetic Dietary and Renal Rickets
1.2.2.5	Scurvy (metaphyseal chip fractures)
1.2.2.6	Menkes Kinky Hair Syndrome

1.2.3   Other Rare Fragile Bone Disorders

Multiple fractures consistently occur in several rare disorders in which other stigmata overshadow the bone fragility.

1.2.3.1	Osteopetrosis
1.2.3.2	Pycnodysostosis
1.2.3.3	Mucolipidosis II (I-Cell Disease)
1.2.3.4	Metaphyseal Chondrodysplasia, Jansen Type
1.2.3.5	Homocystinuria
1.2.3.6	Glycogen Storage Disease
1.2.3.7	Osteolyses (various types)
1.2.3.8	Metaphyseal Dysplasia Sutcliffe Type (corner fractures)
1.2.3.9	Skeletal Dysplasias with Gracile Bones

1.2.4   Skeletal Disorders in Which Fractures Sometimes Occur

In a number of genetic or congenital conditions an inconsistent but increased frequency of fractures is the consequence of defective skeletal structure rather than of osteoporosis.

1.2.4.1	Arthrogryposis Syndromes
1.2.4.2	Fibrous Dysplasia Syndromes
1.2.4.3	Enchondromatosis

1.2.5   Skeletal Fractures in Otherwise Normal Bones

1.2.5.1   Battered Child Syndrome
1.2.5.2   Seizures

The "battered child" or "child abuse" syndrome should be included in the differential diagnosis of every skeletal survey that reveals multiple fractures and any type of unusual or rare single fracture.

1.2.6   Lethal Bone Dysplasias with Fragmented Bones

1.2.6.1   Greenberg Dysplasia
1.2.6.2   Dappled Diaphyseal Dysplasia
1.2.6.3   Astley–Kendall Dysplasia

1.2.7   Corner Fractures

Corner fractures are a feature of conditions that form spurs at the medial aspects of the proximal tibial and distal femoral metaphyses. These fractures, which can occur at other metaphyses, are characteristic of the following disorders:

1.2.7.1   Spondylometaphyseal Dysplasia, Sutcliffe type
1.2.7.2   Spondyloepimetaphyseal Dysplasias;
1.2.7.3   Battered Child Syndrome
1.2.7.4   Scurvy
1.2.7.5   Menkes Kinky Hair Syndrome
1.2.7.6   Blount Disease

1.3   Osteosclerosis and Hyperostosis

The sclerosing bone dysplasias are a group of genetic disorders in which abnormal density of the skeleton predominates. In the past they were frequently lumped together as "osteopetrosis" or "Albers–Schönberg disease", but with increasing diagnostic sophistication, they have been delineated as separate entities, with distinctive clinical and radiological stigmata. They are categorised according to the presence or absence of alteration of skeletal contours, with or without excessive bone overgrowth, in addition to increased radiological density.

In the newborn period benign generalised osteopetrosis may lead to diagnostic confusion with other sclerotic bone disorders, specifically osteopetrosis with precocious manifestations.

1.3.1   Osteoscleroses

Increased skeletal density without significant alteration in bony contours.

1.3.1.1	Osteopetrosis with Delayed Manifestations
1.3.1.2	Osteopetrosis with Precocious Manifestations
1.3.1.3	Osteopetrosis, Intermediate AR form
1.3.1.4	Osteopetrosis with Carbonic Anhydrase II Deficiency
1.3.1.5	Pycnodysostosis

1.3.2   Craniotubular Dysplasias

Increased density, especially of the cranium, together with undermodelling of the long bones.

1.3.2.1	Metaphyseal Dysplasia (Pyle Disease)
1.3.2.2	Craniometaphyseal Dysplasia
1.3.2.3	Frontometaphyseal Dysplasia
1.3.2.4	Osteodysplasty (Melnick–Needles Syndrome)
1.3.2.5	Craniodiaphyseal Dysplasia
1.3.2.6	Dysosteosclerosis

1.3.3   Craniotubular Hyperostoses

Bone overgrowth produces increased density and width with alteration in bone contours.

1.3.3.1	Endosteal Hyperostosis – Worth Type (mild)
1.3.3.1	Endosteal Hyperostosis – van Buchem Type (severe)
1.3.3.3	Sclerosteosis
1.3.3.4	Osteoectasia with Hyperphosphatasia
1.3.3.5	Diaphyseal Dysplasia (Camurati–Engelmann Disease)

1.3.4 Miscellaneous Well-recognised Sclerosing Bone Dysplasias

1.3.4.1   Osteopathia Striata with Cranial Sclerosis
1.3.4.2   Oculodento-osseous Dysplasia
1.3.4.3   Osteomesopycnosis

1.3.5 Rare Sclerosing Bone Dysplasias

1.3.5.1   Osteosclerosis (Stanescu Type)
1.3.5.2   Tubular Stenosis (Kenny–Caffey Syndrome)
1.3.5.3   Schwarz–Lelek Syndrome
1.3.5.4   Sclerotic Bone – Dentine Dysplasia Syndrome
1.3.5.5   Axial Osteosclerosis with Bamboo Hair
           (Trichothiodystrophy or Netherton Syndrome)
1.3.5.6   Weismann–Netter–Stuhl Syndrome
           (Toxopachyostéose Diaphysaire Tibio-Péronière)
1.3.5.7   Lenz–Majewski Dysplasia
1.3.5.8   Cerebellar Hypoplasia with Endosteal Hyperostosis

1.3.6 Skeletal Sclerosis in Other Conditions

1.3.6.1   Paget Disease (Osteitis Deformans)
1.3.6.2   Caffey Disease (Idiopathic Cortical Hyperostosis)
1.3.6.3   Idiopathic Hypercalcaemia
1.3.6.4   Vitamin D Poisoning
1.3.6.5   Renal Osteosclerosis
1.3.6.6   Pachydermoperiostosis (Idiopathic Hypertrophic
           Osteoarthropathy)
1.3.6.7   Secondary Hypertrophic Osteoarthropathy
1.3.6.8   Myelosclerosis
1.3.6.9   Oxalosis
1.3.6.10   Recurrent Symmetrical Periostitis
1.3.6.11   Mastocytosis
1.3.6.12   Tuberous Sclerosis
1.3.6.13   Fluorosis
1.3.6.14   Heavy Metal Poisoning

1.3.7   Sclerotic Foci

Calcific streaking, spots or stippling affecting only the epiphyses and apophyses is an important incidental radiographic feature in the newborn and infantile period. It also occurs in a few rare disorders, several of which are lethal. More extensive stippling and streaking occur throughout the skeleton in a number of bone dysplasias, including several of those listed in previous sections of this chapter. Neoplastic metastases enter into the differential diagnosis of sclerotic foci especially if their distribution is asymmetrical.

Neonates and Infants

1.3.7.1	Chondrodysplasia Punctata
1.3.7.2	Warfarin Embryopathy
1.3.7.3	Cerebro-hepato-renal Syndrome of Zellweger
1.3.7.4	GMI Gangliosidosis
1.3.7.5	Smith–Lemli–Opitz Syndrome
1.3.7.6	De Barsy Syndrome
1.3.7.7	Chromosomal Disorders
1.3.7.8	Binder Syndrome (Maxillofacial Dysplasia)
1.3.7.9	Mucolipidosis II (I-cell Disease)
1.3.7.10	Pacman Dysplasia
1.3.7.11	Spondyloepimetaphyseal Dysplasia, Short Limb Abnormal Calcification Type

Older Children and Adults

1.3.7.12	Osteopoikilosis
1.3.7.13	Melorheostosis
1.3.7.14	Tuberous Sclerosis
1.3.7.15	Osteogenesis Imperfecta
1.3.7.16	Parastremmatic Dysplasia
1.3.7.17	Metaphyseal Chondrodysplasia, Jansen Type
1.3.7.18	Mastocytosis
1.3.7.19	Bone Islands
1.3.7.20	Chondrodysplasia Punctata (mild forms)
1.3.7.21	Sponastrime Dysplasia (striated metaphyses)

1.3.8   Neonatal Severe Osteosclerotic Dysplasia

1.3.8.1	Blomstrand Dysplasia
1.3.8.2	Raine Dysplasia
1.3.8.3	Caffey Disease, Prenatal Onset

1.3.8.4   Dysplastic Cortical Hyperostosis
1.3.8.5   Desmosterolosis (Raine Dysplasia Variant?)

1.4   Periosteal Thickening and Periostitis

Periosteal thickening and periostitis are common manifestations of many different skeletal lesions; they are not uncommon in bone dysplasias and their radiographic recognition raises a wide range of diagnostic possibilities.

1.4.1   Bone Dysplasias

1.4.1.1   Pachydermoperiostosis (Idiopathic Hypertrophic Osteoarthropathy)
1.4.1.2   Diaphyseal Dysplasia (Camurati–Engelmann Disease)
1.4.1.3   Neurofibromatosis (von Recklinghausen Disease) [subperiosteal haemorrhages]
1.4.1.4   Fibrous Dysplasia (McCune–Albright Type)

1.4.2   Other Bone Diseases

1.4.2.1   Caffey Disease (Idiopathic Cortical Hyperostosis)
1.4.2.2   Recurrent Symmetrical Periostitis
1.4.2.3   Paget Disease (Osteitis Deformans)

1.4.3   Traumatic

1.4.3.1   Birth Trauma
1.4.3.2   Manipulation of Newborns and Infants
1.4.3.3   Battered Child Syndrome
1.4.3.4   Neurogenic Disorders (Meningomyelocele, Congenital Insensitivity to Pain, Spinal Cord Damage)
1.4.3.5   Haemophilia

1.4.4   Infection

1.4.4.1   Bacterial Osteomyelitis

1.4.4.2   Syphilis
1.4.4.3   Tuberculosis

1.4.5   Hypo/Hypervitaminosis

1.4.5.1   Rickets (Vitamin D Deficiency)
1.4.5.2   Scurvy (Vitamin C Deficiency; subperiosteal haemorrhage)
1.4.5.3   Hypervitaminosis A
1.4.5.4   Hypervitaminosis D

1.4.6   Skin Disorders

1.4.6.1   Pachydermoperiostosis (Idiopathic Hypertrophic Osteoarthropathy)
1.4.6.2   Ichthyosis Congenita
1.4.6.3   Urticaria Pigmentosa
1.4.6.4   Pyodermia
1.4.6.5   Burns
1.4.6.6   Frostbite
1.4.6.7   Chronic Cellulitis
1.4.6.8   Varicose Ulceration

1.4.7   Tumours

1.4.7.1   Primary Bone Tumours (Ewing Sarcoma, Osteosarcoma, Osteoid Osteoma)
1.4.7.2   Leukaemia
1.4.7.3   Bone Metastasis (Neuroblastoma)
1.4.7.4   Histiocytosis X (Langerhans cell tumour) [especially in infants and small children]
1.4.7.5   Histiocytic Medullary Reticulosis
1.4.7.6   Angio-osteohypertrophy (Klippel–Trenaunay–Weber Syndrome)
1.4.7.7   Erdheim–Chester Disease

1.4.8   Metabolic Disorders

1.4.8.1   Infantile Nutritional Copper Deficiency
1.4.8.2   Hyperphosphatasia

1.4.8.3   Hyperparathyroidism
1.4.8.4   Prostaglandin-induced "Periostitis"
1.4.8.5   Pancreatitis

1.4.9   Miscellaneous

1.4.9.1   Arthritis
1.4.9.2   Acromegaly
1.4.9.3   Tuberous Sclerosis
1.4.9.4   Physiological Periosteal Thickening of the Newborn
1.4.9.5   Hypertrophic Osteoarthropathy, secondary to:
           Congenital Heart Disease
           Bronchiectasis
           Chronic Pneumonia
           Malignancies (Hodgkin disease and other
           lymphomas, carcinomas, other tumours)
           Hepatic Cirrhosis
           Mucoviscidosis
1.4.9.6   Increased Osteoclastic Activity (reflecting rapid
           demineralisation stimulating periostitis)

1.5   Exostoses

Exostoses are a diagnostic sign in some bone dysplasias and congenital
syndromes and represent a clue to recognition in others. Periosteal
excrescences and spurs are included in this category as it may be
impossible to differentiate them from true exostoses.

1.5.1   Generalised Exostoses

1.5.1.1   Multiple Cartilaginous Exostoses (Diaphyseal Aclasis)
1.5.1.2   Trichorhinophalangeal Syndrome Type II (Langer–
           Giedion)
1.5.1.3   Metachondromatosis (hands, feet, knees)
1.5.1.4   Interstitial Deletion of Chromosome 11

1.5.2   Localised Exostoses

1.5.2.1	Solitary Ecchondroma
1.5.2.2	Fibrodysplasia Ossificans Progressiva
1.5.2.3	Dyschondrosteosis (proximal tibiae)
1.5.2.4	Dysplasia Epiphysealis Hemimelica (unilateral, epiphyses affected)
1.5.2.5	Chondroectodermal Dysplasia (Ellis–van Creveld Syndrome, tibia)
1.5.2.6	Osteo-onychodysplasia (iliac horns)
1.5.2.7	Turner Syndrome (proximal tibiae)
1.5.2.8	Pseudohypoparathyroidism. Pseudopseudohypoparathyroidism (Albright Hereditary Osteodystrophy)
1.5.2.9	Acrodysostosis (proximal tibiae)
1.5.2.10	Arteriohepatic Dysplasia
1.5.2.11	Supracondylar Process (humerus)
1.5.2.12	Gardner Syndrome (osteomas)
1.5.2.13	Occipital Horn Syndrome (occipital bony protuberances)

Reactive, degenerative, or hypertrophic spurs (osteophytes) of different aetiology may occur in a variety of anatomical localisations. These acquired abnormalities enter into the differential diagnosis of genetic or syndromic exostoses.

1.6   Multiple Radiolucent Defects

Multiple radiolucent cyst-like defects are an important and potentially serious sign in patients with bone disorders. In essence, the differential diagnosis rests between neoplasia, infection, and a bone dysplasia; other conditions are rarely implicated.

If skeletal survey is available and the clinical history is known, the majority of cystic bone dysplasias can be recognised without biopsy. However, this procedure is often necessary for confirmation and exact diagnosis in a neoplastic process.

1.6.1   Bone Dysplasias

1.6.1.1	Fibrous Dysplasia [Polyostotic] (Jaffe–Lichtenstein Syndrome)

1.6.2   Bone Tumours and Tumour-like Conditions

1.6.3   Miscellaneous

1.7 Advanced and Retarded Bone Age

Advanced and retarded bone age are important radiographic signs. In the first years of life, the optimal views for the appraisal of bone age are lateral and antero-posterior projections (AP) of the foot and postero-anterior projections (PA) of the hands. In later childhood, PA views of the hands are usually adequate, but if more exact bone age estimation is required, AP and lateral radiographs of the feet and AP and lateral radiographs of the knees should be obtained. In the adolescent period, differences in the hand radiographs are slight and thus difficult to evaluate. For this reason estimation of bone age at the elbow is more informative.

In children of school age, advanced or retarded bone age ± 1 year is within normal limits. Variation by up to 2 years either way may still be within normal limits taking into account idiopathic, familial, ethnic, nutritional and other influences together with the reporting radiologist's individuality or idiosyncrasy! Advancement or retardation beyond 2 years should be regarded as abnormal and indicative of an absolute requirement for further investigations. Dysharmonic skeletal maturation (phalangeal versus carpal) is a common feature of bone dysplasias and is present in many syndromic associations.

Advance of bone age is much less common than retardation and it presents a difficult problem. In early life, especially in neonates and infants, advanced bone age may be an important sign of bone dysplasia. In these circumstances the changes often have a specific anatomical appearance. In terms of differential diagnosis, it is important that an endocrine disorder should be considered in every age group.

1.7.1 Advanced Bone Age in Infancy

1.7.1.5   Marshall Syndrome
1.7.1.6   Cerebral Gigantism (Sotos Syndrome)
1.7.1.7   Beckwith–Wiedemann Syndrome
1.7.1.8   Desbuquois Syndrome
1.7.1.9   Hyperthyroidism
1.7.1.10 Adreno-genital Syndrome
1.7.1.11 Simpson–Golabi–Behmel syndrome (Gigantism-dysplasia Syndrome)

1.7.2   Advanced Bone Age in the Older Child

1.7.2.1   Acrodysostosis
1.7.2.2   Fibrous Dysplasia (McCune–Albright Syndrome)
1.7.2.3   Idiopathic Familial Advanced Bone Age
1.7.2.4   Endocrine Disorders

1.7.3   Retarded Bone Age – Severe

1.7.3.1   Hypothyroidism
1.7.3.2   Spondylometaphyseal Dysplasias
1.7.3.3   Spondyloepimetaphyseal Dysplasias

1.7.4   Retarded Bone Age – Moderate to Mild

Moderate to mild retardation of bone age is a non-specific feature of several genetic bone dysplasias, notably the following:

1.7.4.1   Metaphyseal Chondrodysplasia (Shwachman Type)
1.7.4.2   Multiple Epiphyseal Dysplasia
1.7.4.3   Spondylo-epi-metaphyseal Dysplasias (heterogeneous)
1.7.4.4   Spondylometaphyseal Dysplasias (heterogeneous)
1.7.4.5   Cleido-cranial Dysplasia
1.7.4.6   Meyer Dysplasia
1.7.4.7   Osteodysplasty (Melnick–Needles Syndrome)

1.7.5   Retarded Bone Age in Endocrine Disorders

1.7.5.1   Hypothyroidism
1.7.5.2   Hypopituitarism (primary, many types)

1.7.6   Retarded Bone Age in Chromosomal Abnormalities

1.7.7   Retarded Bone Age in Other Syndromes of Developmental Delay

1.8   Complex Generalised Abnormalities

(Dysostosis Multiplex and Related Disorders)
The radiological term "dysostosis multiplex" implies that all the bones are abnormal in size, shape, and texture, and have some specific features such as hypoplasia of upper lumbar vertebrae, narrowing of the proximal ends of the metacarpals, J-shaped sella, etc. These changes are encountered in different patterns and degrees in complex carbohydrate metabolic disorders, known also as the mucopolysaccharidoses, mucolipidoses, and oligosaccharidoses. Although the diagnosis of disorders in this group is primarily biochemical, many of them can be recognised if full skeletal survey is performed and the case history and clinical findings are available.

1.8.1   Mucopolysaccharidoses

1.8.1.1	MPS 1-H (Hurler)
1.8.1.2	MPS 1-S (Scheie)
1.8.1.3	MPS II (Hunter)
1.8.1.4	MPS III (Sanfilippo)
1.8.1.5	MPS IV (Morquio)
1.8.1.6	MPS VI (Maroteaux–Lamy)
1.8.1.7	MPS VII (β-Glucuronidase Deficiency)
1.8.1.8	Multiple Sulfatase Deficiency
1.8.1.9	Others (not well defined)

1.8.2   Mucolipidoses (Sialidoses)

1.8.2.1	MLS I (Neuraminidase Deficiency)
1.8.2.2	MLS II (I-Cell Disease of Leroy)
1.8.2.3	MLS III (Pseudopolydystrophy of Maroteaux)

1.8.3   Oligosaccharidoses

1.8.3.1	Fucosidosis I
1.8.3.2	Fucosidosis II
1.8.3.3	GM.1 Gangliosidosis
1.8.3.4	Mannosidosis
1.8.3.5	Aspartylglucosaminuria

1.9   Asymmetry (Hemihypertrophy or Hemiatrophy)

1.9.1   Asymmetry with Bone Dysplasia

Asymmetrical shortening or lengthening of limbs is a characteristic feature of several genetic or "idiopathic" bone dysplasias.

1.9.1.1	Chondrodysplasia Punctata
1.9.1.2	Dysplasia Epiphysealis Hemimelica
1.9.1.3	Enchondromatosis (Ollier disease)
1.9.1.4	Enchondromatosis with Haemangiomata (Maffucci Syndrome)

1.9.1.5   Fibrous Dysplasia
1.9.1.6   Proteus Syndrome
1.9.1.7   Melorheostosis
1.9.1.8   Tricho-rhino-phalangeal Syndrome II
1.9.1.9   Exchondromatosis

1.9.2   Asymmetry with Bone Overgrowth in the Absence of Any Gross Localised Lesion

1.9.2.1   Russell–Silver Syndrome
1.9.2.2   Beckwith–Wiedemann Syndrome

1.9.3   Asymmetry with Vascular Malformations

Asymmetry may be the consequence of localised or massive overgrowth of bone and soft tissues in association with vascular or lymphatic anomalies.

1.9.3.1   Angio-osteohypertrophy (Klippel–Trenaunay–Weber Syndrome)
1.9.3.2   Lymphangioma

1.9.4   Asymmetry with Primary Neurocutaneous Syndromes (Central or Peripheral Type)

1.9.4.1   Neurofibromatosis (von Recklinghausen Disease)
1.9.4.2   Tuberous Sclerosis
1.9.4.3   Sturge–Weber Syndrome
1.9.4.4   Lindau–von Hippel Disease
1.9.4.5   Epidural naevus

1.9.5   Asymmetry (Hemihypertrophy) with Tumours

Hemihypertrophy (hemihyperplasia) can occur as an isolated feature in an otherwise normal individual or as a syndromic association. A predisposition to neoplasia is present in several forms of hemihypertrophy, notably Wiedemann–Beckwith syndrome, neurofibromatosis, fibrous dysplasia, epidermal naevus syndrome, multiple exostoses and enchondromatosis. This factor is relevant in the long-term follow-up of affected patients.

1.9.5.1   Renal Neoplasms (Wilms Tumour)
1.9.5.2   Hepatic Neoplasms (Hepatoblastoma)
1.9.5.3   Adrenal Gland Neoplasms (Adrenocortical
          Carcinoma, Adenoma)

1.9.6   Acquired Asymmetry

1.9.6.1   Post-traumatic Asymmetry
1.9.6.2   Associated with Neuromuscular Disease
1.9.6.3   Postinflammatory Asymmetry

1.10   Multiple Dislocations

Single joint dislocations or subluxations which are present at birth or occur in later life are a common finding in many malformation syndromes and are of little diagnostic value. Sporadic idiopathic unilateral dislocation of the hip is by far the most frequent congenital anomaly of this type. Bilateral multiple joint dislocations are much less common, but of great diagnostic importance. In all the syndromes in this category, the hips and elbows are predominantly involved. The dislocations may be the consequence of capsular and ligamentous laxity, bone dysplasia, or both. In the dwarfing skeletal disorders in which the odontoid process is hypoplastic, the additional syndromic component of lax ligaments poses a grave risk of atlanto-axial subluxation leading to quadriplegia or death.

1.10.1   Frequent Dislocations

1.10.1.1   Ehlers–Danlos Syndrome
1.10.1.2   Familial Articular Hypermobility Syndrome
1.10.1.3   Larsen Syndrome
1.10.1.4   Spondylo-epi-metaphyseal Dysplasia with Joint Laxity
           (SEMDJL)
1.10.1.5   Desbuquois Syndrome
1.10.1.6   RAPADILINO Syndrome

1.10.2   Inconsistent Dislocations

Congenital dislocations are an inconsistent feature of certain conditions, some of which are otherwise characterised by joint rigidity. This paradoxical situation is probably the result of defective development of the bony components of the affected joints.

1.10.2.1	Arthrogryposis
1.10.2.2	Diastrophic Dysplasia
1.10.2.3	Pseudodiastrophic Dysplasia
1.10.2.4	Mesomelic Dysplasia (Werner type)
1.10.2.5	Osteogenesis Imperfecta
1.10.2.6	De Barsy Syndrome

1.11   Soft Tissue Calcification

Calcification in the soft tissues is an important sign in several metabolic diseases. Nevertheless, recognition of this abnormality rarely permits accurate diagnosis in the absence of clinical and biochemical investigations. It must be emphasised that the distinction between ectopic calcification and ossification is not always obvious. It is important to establish, with lesions near joints, whether the calcification is in epiphyseal or articular cartilage or in other tissues.

1.11.1   Multifocal Calcification or Ossification in Genetic Disorders

1.11.1.1	Fibrodysplasia Ossificans Progressiva
1.11.1.2	Singleton–Merten Syndrome
1.11.1.3	Pseudohypoparathyroidism, Pseudopseudohypoparathyroidism (Albright Hereditary Osteodystrophy)
1.11.1.4	Tumoral Calcinosis
1.11.1.5	Hypophosphatasia
1.11.1.6	Menkes Kinky Hair Syndrome
1.11.1.7	Rothmund–Thompson Syndrome

1.11.2   Localised Calcification or Ossification in Genetic Disorders

1.11.2.1   Diastrophic Dysplasia (pinna calcification)
1.11.2.2   Ehlers–Danlos Syndrome (subcutaneous spheroids)
1.11.2.3   Keutel Syndrome (tracheal calcification)
1.11.2.4   Chondrodysplasia Punctata (epiphyseal, periarticular, tarsal bone anlage, laryngo-tracheo-bronchial)
1.11.2.5   Singleton–Merten Syndrome (thoracic aorta)

1.11.3   Acquired forms of Generalised or Localised Ectopic Calcification

1.11.3.1   Myositis Ossificans (frequently not actually in muscle)
1.11.3.2   Collagen Disorders (Dermatomyositis, Scleroderma, Lupus Erythematosis)
1.11.3.3   Metabolic Disorders (Renal and Parathyroid Dysfunction)
1.11.3.4   Parasitic Diseases (Filariasis, Guinea Worm, Hydatid Cysts)
1.11.3.5   Vascular (Calcified Vessels, Phleboliths)
1.11.3.6   Renal Transplantation
1.11.3.7   Extravasation of Calcium Gluconate

1.12   Skeletal Dysplasia in the Newborn

The presence of a generalised skeletal dysplasia in a stillborn or newborn infant poses special problems in radiological practice. Although conditions in this category are individually rare, collectively they are not uncommon. Many generalised bone dysplasias are clinically apparent in the neonate, but in the majority the final diagnosis is dependent on radiological studies. New conditions of this type continue to be delineated and in order to avoid confusion, excessively rare or ill-defined disorders have been omitted from this section.

The nature of the specific disorder will influence prognostication, genetic measures, and the obstetrical management of further pregnancies. For these reasons, diagnostic precision is crucial. Indeed, it has been suggested that diagnostic radiological investigations are indicated in any stillborn child, and in this context it is significant that excellent radiographs can be obtained from a deceased neonate.

The conditions in question, as listed below, have been categorised according to their compatibility with life. It must be emphasised, however, that although these broad generalisations hold true, exceptions occur in individual cases.

1.12.1 Lethal

1.12.1.1	Thanatophoric Dysplasia
1.12.1.2	Thanatophoric Dysplasia with Cloverleaf Skull
1.12.1.3	Achondrogenesis (several types)
1.12.1.4	Short Rib Syndrome (several types)
1.12.1.5	Homozygous Achondroplasia
1.12.1.6	Fibrochondroplasia
1.12.1.7	Atelosteogenesis (several types)
1.12.1.8	Hypochondrogenesis
1.12.1.9	Hypophosphatasia (severe type)
1.12.1.10	Boomerang Dysplasia
1.12.1.11	Spondylodysplastic Perinatally Lethal Group (San Diego, Torrence, Luton types)
1.12.1.12	Opsismodysplasia

1.12.2 Potentially Lethal

1.12.2.1	Chondrodysplasia Punctata – Rhizomelic Form
1.12.2.2	Campomelic Dysplasia
1.12.2.3	Asphyxiating Thoracic Dysplasia (Jeune Syndrome)
1.12.2.4	Osteogenesis Imperfecta Type II
1.12.2.5	Osteopetrosis with Precocious Manifestations
1.12.2.6	Dyssegmental Dysplasia
1.12.2.7	Oto-palato-digital Syndrome II

1.12.3 Viable

1.12.3.1	Achondroplasia
1.12.3.2	SADDAN Dysplasia (severe achondroplasia, developmental delay, acanthosis nigricans)
1.12.3.3	Chondrodysplasia Punctata – Dominant Form
1.12.3.4	Diastrophic Dysplasia
1.12.3.5	Metatropic Dysplasia

1.12.3.6	Kniest Dysplasia
1.12.3.7	Chondroectodermal Dysplasia (Ellis–van Creveld)
1.12.3.8	Spondyloepiphyseal Dysplasia Congenita
1.12.3.9	Spondylo-epi-metaphyseal Dysplasia Congenita
1.12.3.10	Mesomelic Dysplasias
1.12.3.11	Acromesomelic Dysplasia
1.12.3.13	Larsen Syndrome
1.12.3.14	Spondylocostal Dysostosis (Spondylothoracic Dysplasia)
1.12.3.15	Cleidocranial Dysplasia

1.12.4   Neonatal Severe Osteosclerotic Dysplasias

1.12.4.1	Blomstrand Dysplasia
1.12.4.2	Raine Dysplasia
1.12.4.3	Prenatal Onset Caffey Disease
1.12.4.4	Dysplastic Cortical Hyperostosis

1.13   Premature Ageing Syndromes

More than 30 premature ageing syndromes have been recognised. Some of them, such as the Wiedemann–Rautenstrauch syndrome are present at birth, whereas others such as progeria develop during the first few years of life. Although radiographic findings are seldom diagnostic, a full skeletal survey is obligatory as it may help to confirm or negate the diagnosis of a specific form of a premature ageing syndrome.

1.13.1	Growth Hormone Deficiency Syndromes
1.13.2	Geroderma Osteodysplastica
1.13.3	Progeria and other Progeroid Syndromes
1.13.4	Hallermann–Streiff Syndrome
1.13.5	Leprechaunism
1.13.6	Wiedemann–Rautenstrauch Syndrome (see Progeria)
1.13.7	Lenz–Majewski Dysplasia
1.13.8	Taybi–Linder Syndrome (Cephaloskeletal Dysplasia)
1.13.9	De Barsy Syndrome
1.13.10	Cockayne Syndrome
1.13.11	Cutis Laxa Syndrome
1.13.12	Acrogeria (hands and feet)
1.13.13	Mandibulo-acral Dysostosis
1.13.14	Mulvihill–Smith Syndrome

Section 2

Regional Skeletal Abnormalities

2.1   Skull

2.1.1   Abnormal Configuration of the Skull

2.1.1.1   Craniostenosis
2.1.1.2   Microcephaly
2.1.1.3   Macrocephaly

2.1.2   Increased Density of the Skull

2.1.2.1   Osteosclerosis
2.1.2.2   Craniotubular Dysplasias
2.1.2.3   Craniotubular Hyperostoses
2.1.2.4   Miscellaneous

2.1.3   Defective Cranial Development and/or Ossification

2.1.3.1   Delayed Closure of Sutures or Fontanels
2.1.3.2   Wormian Bones
2.1.3.3   Bony Expansion of the Calvarium
2.1.3.4   Persistent Parietal Foramen

2.1.4   Intracranial Calcification

2.1.4.1   Bone Dysplasias
2.1.4.2   Infections
2.1.4.3   Metabolic Disorders
2.1.4.4   Endocrine Disorders
2.1.4.5   Other Disorders

2.1.5   Miscellaneous Cranial Abnormalities

2.1.5.1   Sella Turcica Abnormalities
2.1.5.2   Abnormal Facial Structures

2.1.6   Mandibular and Dental Abnormalities

2.1.6.1   Mandibular Configuration
2.1.6.2   Fibrocystic Lesions of the Mandible
2.1.6.3   Dental Abnormalities

2.1.1 Abnormal Configuration of the Skull

2.1.1.1 Craniostenosis

Premature fusion of cranial sutures produces alteration in the shape of the head. Terms that are conventionally applied to specific configurations are explained below.

Scaphocephaly or Dolichocephaly	A boat-shaped or long narrow skull
Acrocephaly	A sharp or superiorly pointed skull
Oxycephaly or Turricephaly	A skull with increased vertical diameter and reduced AP and lateral diameters; a tower-shaped head
Plagiocephaly	An asymmetrical twisted skull
Trigonocephaly	An anteriorly pointed skull
Brachycephaly	A skull reduced in the AP diameter
Cloverleaf skull	A skull with anterior constrictions producing a trilobal configuration

Craniostenosis often occurs in isolation, when it produces a generally small head, with a normal shape. More frequently, involvement of only one or two sutures leads to asymmetry of the skull. Craniostenosis is also a significant component of several important syndromes in which the actual shape of the head is variable.

2.1.1.1.1 *Craniostenosis with Digital Abnormalities*
Apert Syndrome (Acrocephalosyndactyly)
Carpenter Syndrome (Acrocephalopolysyndactyly)
Other Rare Acrocephalosyndactyly and Acrocephalopolysyndactyly Syndromes
Craniosynostosis with Radial Defects (Baller–Gerold Syndrome)

2.1.1.1.2 *Other conditions in which craniostenosis is a component*
Chromosomal Disorders
Hypophosphatasia
Idiopathic Hypercalcaemia
Idiopathic Hypercalciuria
Hyperthyroidism

2.1.1.1.3 *Cloverleaf Skull*
Thanatophoric Dysplasia II (straight femur type)
Osteoglophonic Dysplasia
Campomelic Dysplasia
Isolated Clover Leaf Skull

2.1.1.2   Microcephaly

Microcephaly or small cranium can be best appreciated by physical examination and measurement, with reference to standard developmental charts. Microcephaly has little value in the diagnosis of the skeletal dysplasias unless it is associated with additional abnormalities such as premature closure of cranial sutures, defective skull ossification, or brain abnormalities as detected on computerised tomography (CT) or magentic resonance (MR) scanning. Microcephaly is a common finding in syndromes in which mental retardation is associated with multiple anomalies.

2.1.1.3   Macrocephaly

Macrocephaly or large cranium is present in many syndromes and it has diagnostic importance if additional radiographic signs such as wormian bones or widened sutures are also present. Sometimes apparent macrocephaly is spurious in that the cranium seems to be large in relation to a small face, as in cleidocranial dysplasia, the Russell–Silver syndrome, and pycnodysostosis.

Macrocephaly occurs in the following genetic disorders:

> 2.1.1.3.1   *Achondroplasia*
> 2.1.1.3.2   *Hurler Syndrome (MPS I-H)*
> 2.1.1.3.3   *Osteogenesis Imperfecta*
> 2.1.1.3.4   *Cerebral Gigantism (Sotos Syndrome)*
> 2.1.1.3.5   *Tubular Stenosis (Kenny–Caffey Syndrome)*
> 2.1.1.3.6   *Neurofibromatosis (von Recklinghausen Disease)*
> 2.1.1.3.7   *Pycnodysostosis*
> 2.1.1.3.8   *Cleidocranial Dysplasia*
> 2.1.1.3.9   *Osteopathia striata with cranial sclerosis*
> 2.1.1.3.10 *Hajdu–Cheney syndrome*

Macrocephaly is also the consequence of hydrocephaly, which may be communicating or non-communicating. This condition may result from congenital malformation of the brain, or in association with neural tube defects. Important acquired causes of hydrocephaly include meningitis, intracranial haemorrhage and cerebral tumours; rarely it may be idiopathic.

2.1.2   Increased Density of the Skull

Increased density and/or hyperostosis of the skull base and calvarium are present in the sclerosing bone dysplasias. In the majority, the skeletal changes are generalised, and on the basis of the distribution and configuration of these abnormalities, this group of conditions is conventionally subclassified into the osteoscleroses, craniotubular dysplasias, and craniotubular hyperostoses.

In conditions of this type, basal sclerosis may be present without significant calvarial involvement, but the converse rarely occurs. A distinction between sclerosis (i.e. increase in bone density without alteration in width) and hyperostosis (i.e. bone overgrowth leading to increase in density and width) is often of diagnostic significance, but it must be appreciated that some cases do not fit neatly into either category. It is also of importance that the radiological changes are age related, and that definitive diagnosis may be difficult in early childhood.

2.1.2.1 Osteoscleroses

Increased bone density without significant alteration in skeletal contours.

> 2.1.2.1.1 *Osteopetrosis (infantile type)*
> 2.1.2.1.2 *Osteopetrosis (delayed-onset type)*
> 2.1.2.1.3 *Osteopetrosis with carbonic anhydrase II deficiency*
> 2.1.2.1.4 *Osteopetrosis, intermediate type*
> 2.1.2.1.5 *Pycnodysostosis*
> 2.1.2.1.6 *Benign Osteosclerosis of Infancy (transient)*
> 2.1.2.1.7 *Osteopathia Striata with Cranial Sclerosis*

2.1.2.2 Craniotubular Dysplasias

Increased skull density with abnormal modelling of the long bones.

> 2.1.2.2.1 *Metaphyseal Dysplasia (Pyle Disease)*
> 2.1.2.2.2 *Craniometaphyseal Dysplasia*
> 2.1.2.2.3 *Craniodiaphyseal Dysplasia*
> 2.1.2.2.4 *Frontometaphyseal Dysplasia*
> 2.1.2.2.5 *Osteodysplasty (Melnick–Needles Syndrome)*
> 2.1.2.2.6 *Dysosteosclerosis*
> 2.1.2.2.7 *Oculodento-osseous Dysplasia*
> 2.1.2.2.8 *Craniometaphyseal Dysplasia, Wormian Bone Type*

2.1.2.3 Craniotubular Hyperostoses

Increased bone density and width due to overgrowth.

> 2.1.2.3.1 *Endosteal Hyperostosis – Severe van Buchem Type*
> 2.1.2.3.2 *Endosteal Hyperostosis – Mild Worth Type*
> 2.1.2.3.3 *Sclerosteosis*
> 2.1.2.3.4 *Diaphyseal Dysplasia (Camurati–Engelmann Disease)*
> 2.1.2.3.5 *Osteoectasia (Hyperphosphatasia)*

2.1.2.4   Miscellaneous

All conditions that cause generalised osteosclerosis affect the skull.
Predominant or localised sclerosis of the base of the skull occurs in fibrous dysplasia, metaphyseal chondrodysplasia-type Jansen, severe anaemia, hypercalciuria, and Paget disease. It may also be of neoplastic
(meningioma) or inflammatory origin. Hyperostosis frontalis interna is a
common finding in middle-aged women. Local overgrowth of the supraorbital ridges of the frontal bones is a diagnostic feature of frontometaphyseal dysplasia.

2.1.3   Defective Cranial Development and/or Ossification

2.1.3.1   Delayed Closure of Sutures or Fontanels

The recognition of defective and/or delayed calvarial ossification is important in the radiographic diagnosis of bone dysplasias. Although some
features of delayed ossification, such as delay of closure of the anterior
fontanel, can be recognised clinically, radiographic examination gives a
much better overview.

   Defective cranial ossification is characterised by large fontanels, wide
sutures, retarded ossification of the calvarium, and the presence of
wormian bones. It is a hallmark of several bone dysplasias, as well as other
disorders.

> *2.1.3.1.1   Osteogenesis Imperfecta*
> *2.1.3.1.2   Cleidocranial Dysplasia*
> *2.1.3.1.3   Hypothyroidism*
> *2.1.3.1.4   Hypophosphatasia*
> *2.1.3.1.5   Osteodysplasty (Melnick–Needles Syndrome)*
> *2.1.3.1.6   Pycnodysostosis*
> *2.1.3.1.7   Cerebro-hepato-renal Syndrome (Zellweger)*
> *2.1.3.1.8   Russell–Silver Syndrome*
> *2.1.3.1.9   Oculo-mandibulo-facial Syndrome (Hallermann–*
> *   Streiff)*
> *2.1.3.1.10 Mental Retardation – Multiple Anomalies Syndromes*

Cranial ossification is defective in metabolic disorders such as rickets
(dietary, vitamin D-resistant, and renal), in certain chromosomal conditions, notably trisomy 13, and as a normal variant (parietal foramina).

2.1.3.2   Wormian Bones

The presence of a few wormian bones is usually regarded as a normal variant, but multiple wormian bones are an important sign in the disorders listed below:

2.1.3.2.1   *Osteogenesis Imperfecta*
2.1.3.2.2   *Cleidocranial Dysplasia*
2.1.3.2.3   *Hypothyroidism*
2.1.3.2.4   *Pycnodysostosis*

Wormian bones are present but of secondary diagnostic importance in many other disorders, notably:

2.1.3.2.5   *Chromosomal Syndromes*
2.1.3.2.6   *Acro-osteolysis Syndromes (notably Hajdu–Cheney Syndrome)*
2.1.3.2.7   *Oto-palato-digital Syndrome*
2.1.3.2.8   *Oculo-mandibulo-facial Syndrome (Hallermann–Streiff)*
2.1.3.2.9   *Progeria*
2.1.3.2.10   *Pachydermoperiostosis (Idiopathic Hypertrophic Osteoarthropathy)*
2.1.3.2.11   *Cerebro-hepato-renal Syndrome (Zellweger)*
2.1.3.2.12   *Prader–Willi Syndrome*
2.1.3.2.13   *Infantile Nutritional Copper Deficiency*
2.1.3.2.14   *Menkes Kinky Hair Syndrome*
2.1.3.2.15   *Hypophosphatasia*
2.1.3.2.16   *Aminopterin Embryopathy*
2.1.3.2.17   *Craniometaphyseal dysplasia, Wormian Bone Type*
2.1.3.2.18   *Osteodysplasty (Melnick–Needles Syndrome)*

Wormian bones are also encountered in ill-defined syndromes involving mental retardation with multiple anomalies, but in these circumstances their presence is of doubtful diagnostic significance.

2.1.3.3   Bony Expansion of the Calvarium

Expansion of the bones of the cranial vault is a non-specific, although sometimes very obvious radiological sign. Conditions characterised by expansion in association with increased density (i.e. hyperostosis) have been listed in 2.1.2. In addition, calvarial expansion with varying degrees of sclerosis occurs in the following disorders:

2.1.3.3.1   *Bone Marrow Hyperplasia (Anaemias)*
2.1.3.3.2   *Hypoparathyroidism*
2.1.3.3.3   *Pseudohypoparathyroidism (Albright Hereditary Osteodystrophy)*

Calvarial expansion may be present in microcephaly that is secondary to decreased brain growth or brain damage, and in a few rare disorders including acrodysostosis and the Cockayne syndrome.

2.1.3.4   Persistent Parietal Foramen

> 2.1.3.4.1   *Anatomical variant, dominantly inherited*
> 2.1.3.4.2   *Interstitial deletion of chromosome 11p*
> 2.1.3.4.3   *Rare sporadic syndromic associations*

2.1.4   Intracranial Calcification

Intracranial calcification is seldom of diagnostic importance in the bone dysplasias. It may, however, be helpful in directing investigations into the proper channels, depending on the anatomical distribution of the changes. Intracranial calcification is much earlier and better demonstrated by CT than by conventional radiography. It is noteworthy that CT reveals that "physiological" intracranial calcification is a very frequent finding in adults.

Non-physiological intracranial calcification may be present in the following circumstances:

2.1.4.1   Bone Dysplasias

> 2.1.4.1.1   *Basal Cell Naevus Carcinoma Syndrome*
> 2.1.4.1.2   *Oculodento-osseous Dysplasia*
> 2.1.4.1.3   *Tubular Stenosis (Kenny–Caffey Syndrome)*
> 2.1.4.1.4   *Cockayne Syndrome*
> 2.1.4.1.5   *Spondyloenchondromatosis with basal ganglia calcifications*

2.1.4.2   Infections

> 2.1.4.2.1   *Meningo-encephalitis (Herpes Simplex, Toxoplasmosis, Tuberculosis, Cytomegalic Inclusion Disease, etc.)*

2.1.4.3   Metabolic Disorders

> 2.1.4.3.1   *Hypercalcaemia*
> 2.1.4.3.2   *Hypervitaminosis D*
> 2.1.4.3.3   *Homocystinuria*
> 2.1.4.3.4   *Osteopetrosis with Carbonic Anhydrase II Deficiency*

2.1.4.4   Endocrine Disorders

2.1.4.4.1   Idiopathic Hyperparathyroidism
2.1.4.4.2   Hypoparathyroidism
2.1.4.4.3   Pseudohypoparathyroidism (Albright Hereditary
Osteodystrophy)

2.1.4.5   Other Disorders

2.1.4.5.1   Toxic or Anoxic Conditions
2.1.4.5.2   Premature Ageing Syndromes
2.1.4.5.3   Neuroectodermal Syndromes
2.1.4.5.4   Cerebro-oculo-facio-skeletal Syndrome
Pena–Shokeir)
2.1.4.5.5   Others

Intracranial calcifications associated with neoplasms, notably craniophar-yngiomata, gliomata, or meningiomata, are of the utmost diagnostic im-portance. In addition, intracranial calcification may result from intracranial haemorrhage, from anticancer therapy, as a late effect of radiation, or following intoxication with lead or carbon monoxide. Finally, intracranial calcification can be simulated as an artifact by the external application of paste used for electroencephalographic studies.

2.1.5   Miscellaneous Cranial Abnormalities

2.1.5.1   Sella Turcica Abnormalities

An enlarged or abnormally shaped pituitary fossa is an important, although non-specific, radiographic sign. This abnormality always necessitates exclusion of the possibility of a tumour, especially if it is accompanied by intracranial calcification. Enlargement of the sella turcica also occurs in hydrocephalus and in the empty sella syndrome. (The syndromic status of this latter abnormality is uncertain.)

A J-shaped pituitary fossa is a frequent finding in the mucopolysacchar-idoses (MPS). This configuration may also be a normal variant or a component of trisomy 18.

2.1.5.2   Abnormal Facial Structures

Radiographic changes in the facial bones are of little value in the diagnosis of the inherited bone dysplasias. Indeed, abnormalities of the facial structures, including hypertelorism, saddle nose, and bossing of the forehead, are better appreciated on clinical examination than on radio-graphic studies. This latter approach, however, is of importance in assessment prior to reconstructive surgery.

2.1.6   Mandibular and Dental Abnormalities

2.1.6.1   Mandibular Configuration

2.1.6.1.1   Hypoplasia

Significant mandibular hypoplasia that occurs in isolation is termed the "Pierre Robin anomaly". Micrognathia is also a feature of numerous conditions that are diagnosed on a basis of additional syndromic stigmata. The most common and important of these disorders are:

> Treacher Collins Syndrome (Mandibulofacial Dysostosis)
> Goldenhar Syndrome
> Arthro-ophthalmopathy (Stickler Syndrome)
> Mandibulo-acral Dysplasia

2.1.6.1.2   Increased Mandibular Angle

An increased or obtuse mandibular angle is a significant feature of pycnodysostosis. It is not an important component of any other syndrome, but it has been reported in the oto-palato-digital syndrome, metaphyseal dysplasia (Pyle disease), oculodento-osseous dysplasia, and acrodysostosis. In these disorders however this feature is overshadowed by the other skeletal manifestations.

2.1.6.1.3   Prognathism

Mandibular prognathism is a major manifestation of several sclerosing bone dysplasias, notably van Buchem disease and sclerosteosis. Diagnosis is dependent on the recognition of changes in other regions of the skeleton in these conditions.

2.1.6.2   Cystic Lesions of the Mandible

Mandibular cysts and fibrocystic lesions are of little diagnostic value in the bone dysplasias. They may, however, be a valuable sign in the naevoid basal cell carcinoma syndrome and some other very rare conditions.

> 2.1.6.2.1   Basal Cell Naevus Carcinoma Syndrome
> 2.1.6.2.2   Cherubism
> 2.1.6.2.3   Gardner Syndrome
> 2.1.6.2.4   Dental Cysts (Congenital and Inflammatory)
> 2.1.6.2.5   Tumours

2.1.6.3 Dental Abnormalities

Abnormalities of the teeth can best be demonstrated by orthopantomo-graphy (panorex) films. Although important in orthodontics, dental changes are of little value in differential diagnosis of skeletal dysplasias.

2.1.6.3.1 Unerupted Teeth

Failure or delay in eruption of the teeth is a feature of several genetic syndromes, the most important of which is anhydrotic ectodermal dysplasia. Dental delay also occurs in hypopituitarism and hypothyroid-ism.

2.1.6.3.2 Dentinogenesis Imperfecta

This condition presents with an opalescent brownish or purple discolor-ation of the teeth. It can occur as an isolated autosomal dominant entity or as a component of osteogenesis imperfecta.

2.2   Spine

2.2.1   Spinal Malalignment

2.2.1.1   Kyphoscoliosis with Generalised Vertebral Abnormalities
2.2.1.2   Kyphoscoliosis with Localised Vertebral Abnormality
2.2.1.3   Thoracolumbar Wedging
2.2.1.4   Cervical Spine Kyphosis with Generalised Bone Dysplasia

2.2.2   Vertebral Malformation or Deformity

2.2.2.1   Characteristic Shape of the Vertebral Bodies
2.2.2.2   Generalised Platyspondyly – Severe
2.2.2.3   Generalised Platyspondyly – Moderate to Mild
2.2.2.4   Anisospondyly
2.2.2.5   Vertebra Plana
2.2.2.6   Tall Vertebral Bodies

2.2.3   Vertebral Malsegmentation or Fusion

2.2.3.1   Malsegmentation
2.2.3.2   Fusion

2.2.4   Vertebral Abnormalities – Miscellaneous

2.2.4.1   Coronal Clefts
2.2.4.2   Scalloping
2.2.4.3   Odontoid Hypoplasia
2.2.4.4   Interpediculate Narrowing
2.2.4.5   Widening of the Spinal Canal
2.2.4.6   Sagittal Clefts (Butterfly Vertebrae)

2.2.5   Calcification of the Intervertebral Discs

2.2.5.1   Genetic or Congenital Disorders
2.2.5.2   Acquired Conditions

2.2.1   Spinal Malalignment

Severe, progressive kyphoscoliosis is a significant complication in several bone dysplasias. In some of these conditions it occurs with consistency and progresses in spite of early treatment, ultimately causing serious disability. Kyphoscoliosis can also complicate the inherited connective tissue disorders, notably the Ehlers–Danlos syndrome and familial articular hypermobility, in which the skeleton is not primarily involved. It must be emphasised that idiopathic scoliosis, which develops in the absence of any primary vertebral abnormality, is by far the most common form of spinal malalignment.

2.2.1.1   Kyphoscoliosis with Generalised Vertebral Abnormalities

> *2.2.1.1.1   Spondylo-epiphyseal Dysplasia Congenita*
> *2.2.1.1.2   Spondylo-epi-metaphyseal Dysplasia (Heterogeneous)*
> *2.2.1.1.3   Spondylo-epi-metaphyseal Dysplasia with Joint Laxity and Severe Progressive Kyphoscoliosis (SEMDJL)*
> *2.2.1.1.4   Pseudoachondroplasia*
> *2.2.1.1.5   Metatropic Dysplasia*
> *2.2.1.1.6   Diastrophic Dysplasia*
> *2.2.1.1.7   Pseudodiastrophic Dysplasia*
> *2.2.1.1.8   Kniest Dysplasia*
> *2.2.1.1.9   Spondylocostal Dysostosis (Spondylothoracic Dysplasia)*

2.2.1.2   Kyphoscoliosis with Localised Vertebral Abnormality

> *2.2.1.2.1   Neurofibromatosis (von Recklinghausen Disease)*
> *2.2.1.2.2   Hemivertebrae*
> *2.2.1.2.3   Chondrodysplasia Punctata*

2.2.1.3   Thoracolumbar Wedging

This radiographic finding is almost always indicative of a potentially serious disorder and requires further investigations until the cause is established. It is an important feature of the following:

> *2.2.1.3.1   Achondroplasia*
> *2.2.1.3.2   Hypothyroidism*
> *2.2.1.3.3   Disorders of Complex Carbohydrate Metabolism (MPS and MLS)*
> *2.2.1.3.4   Muscular Hypotonia*
> *2.2.1.3.5   Post-traumatic*

2.2.1.4   Cervical Spine Kyphosis with Generalised Bone Dysplasia

In some bone dysplasias with vertebral involvement, the most severe changes are present in the cervical spine. Kyphosis in this region represents an important diagnostic sign in the following:

> *2.2.1.4.1   Neurofibromatosis (von Recklinghausen Disease)*
> *2.2.1.4.2   Larsen Syndrome*
> *2.2.1.4.3   Diastrophic Dysplasia*
> *2.2.1.4.4   Campomelic Dysplasia*
> *2.2.1.4.5   Burton dysplasia*

2.2.2   Vertebral Malformation or Deformity

2.2.2.1   Characteristic Shape of the Vertebral Bodies

In certain skeletal dysplasias, recognition of the characteristic shape of the vertebral bodies is the single most important diagnostic criterion. It is of practical importance that vertebral configuration often changes with age.

> *2.2.2.1.1   Achondroplasia (cuneiform later in life)*
> *2.2.2.1.2   Pseudoachondroplasia (oval with tongue-like projection)*
> *2.2.2.1.3   Mucopolysaccharidoses: specifically Morquio Disease – MPS IV (irregular platyspondyly with anterior tongue-like projection)*
> *2.2.2.1.4   Metatropic dysplasia ("paper thin" in neonates)*
> *2.2.2.1.5   Fibrochondrogenesis (pear-shaped with coronal cleft)*
> *2.2.2.1.6   Thanatophoric Dysplasia (H-shaped in AP projection)*
> *2.2.2.1.7   Spondylo-metaphyseal Dysplasia – Kozlowski Type (elongated anterior tongue-like projection)*
> *2.2.2.1.8   Spondylo-epiphyseal Dysplasia Tarda (hump-shaped)*
> *2.2.2.1.9   Dyggve–Melchior–Clausen Dysplasia (double vertebral hump with central constriction at both vertebral end plates)*
> *2.2.2.1.10 Smith–McCort Syndrome (as in 2.2.2.1.9)*
> *2.2.2.1.11 Opsismodysplasia (paper thin)*
> *2.2.2.1.12 Spondylometaphyseal Dysplasia (Sutcliffe or corner fracture type)*

In a number of disorders the vertebral bodies have an "H-shaped" appearance in lateral views. This configuration is also termed the "step-off" vertebra and it may be encountered in the following:

> Sickle-cell Haemoglobinopathy
> Gaucher Disease

Thalassaemia Major
Hereditary Spherocytosis
Osteoporosis

2.2.2.2   Generalised Platyspondyly – Severe

Generalised platyspondyly is often the most important diagnostic sign in the recognition or exclusion of many bone dysplasias. It may be severe and frequently accompanied by a characteristic shape of the vertebral bodies in the following:

2.2.2.2.1   Osteogenesis Imperfecta (more often Anisospondyly)
2.2.2.2.2   Morquio Disease – MPS IV (platyspondyly increasing with age)
2.2.2.2.3   Spondylo-metaphyseal Dysplasia (various types)
2.2.2.2.4   Metatropic Dysplasia
2.2.2.2.5   Spondylo-epi-metaphyseal Dysplasia (heterogeneous)
2.2.2.2.6   Dyggve–Melchior–Clausen Dysplasia
2.2.2.2.7   Smith–McCort Syndrome
2.2.2.2.8   Parastremmatic Dysplasia
2.2.2.2.9   Thanatophoric Dysplasia
2.2.2.2.10   Achondrogenesis
2.2.2.2.11   Homozygous Achondroplasia
2.2.2.2.12   Brachyolmia (several types)
2.2.2.2.13   Opsismodysplasia
2.2.2.2.14   Long-standing Metabolic Disorders with Osteoporosis (Idiopathic Osteoporosis, Homocystinuria, etc.)
2.2.2.2.15   Lethal platyspondylic skeletal dysplasias (San Diego, Torrance, Luton types)

2.2.2.3   Generalised Platyspondyly – Moderate to Mild

Generalised platyspondyly of moderate to mild degree is common and non-specific; the conditions listed below are those in which the changes are of significant magnitude.

2.2.2.3.1   Spondyloepiphyseal Dysplasia Congenita
2.2.2.3.2   Spondyloepiphyseal Dysplasia Tarda
2.2.2.3.3   Spondylometaphyseal Dysplasia
2.2.2.3.4   Progressive Pseudorheumatoid Dysplasia
2.2.2.3.5   Spondyloepiphyseal Dysplasia with diabetes mellitus (Wolcott–Rallison)
2.2.2.3.6   Pseudoachondroplasia (platyspondyly decreasing with age)
2.2.2.3.7   Dysosteosclerosis (the only sclerotic bone disorder with platyspondyly)
2.2.2.3.8   Achondroplasia (in early life)

2.2.2.3.9   *Myotonic Chondrodysplasia (Schwartz–Jampel Syndrome)*
2.2.2.3.10 *Geroderma Osteodysplastica*
2.2.2.3.11 *Osteogenesis Imperfecta (more often anisospondyly)*
2.2.2.3.12 *Myhre Syndrome*
2.2.2.3.13 *Spondyloenchondrodysplasia*
2.2.2.3.14 *Hypothyroidism*
2.2.2.3.15 *Long-standing Metabolic Disorders with Osteoporosis (Idiopathic Osteoporosis, Homocystinuria, etc.)*

2.2.2.4   Anisospondyly

Irregular flattening of two or more of the vertebral bodies in the presence of other normal vertebrae is termed "anisospondyly". This is a common and important finding in many bone dysplasias.

2.2.2.4.1   *Osteogenesis Imperfecta*
2.2.2.4.2   *Spondylo-epiphyseal Dysplasia (various types)*
2.2.2.4.3   *Spondylo-epi-metaphyseal Dysplasia (various types)*
2.2.2.4.4   *Spondylometaphyseal Dysplasia (various types)*
2.2.2.4.5   *Kniest Dysplasia*
2.2.2.4.6   *Arthro-ophthalmopathy (Stickler Syndrome)*
2.2.2.4.7   *Campomelic Dysplasia*
2.2.2.4.8   *Metabolic Disorders with Osteoporosis (Idiopathic Osteoporosis, Homocystinuria, Steroid Therapy)*
2.2.2.4.9   *Acquired: Trauma, Infection, Irradiation*

2.2.2.5   Vertebra Plana

Vertebra plana (i.e. a single flattened vertebra) is not a sign of bone dysplasia. It may cause some confusion in multifocal histiocytosis X (Langerhans cell tumour) but the aetiologic diagnosis of vertebra plana is normally easy if the case history is available to the radiologist.

2.2.2.5.1   *Histiocytosis X*
2.2.2.5.2   *Tumour (Primary or Secondary)*
2.2.2.5.3   *Trauma*
2.2.2.5.4   *Infection*

2.2.2.6   Tall Vertebral Bodies

Tall vertebral bodies are common in persons with muscular hypotonia and are of little diagnostic value in recognising bone dysplasias. They are seen in the following conditions:

2.2.2.6.1   *Spondylocostal Dysostosis (Spondylothoracic Dysplasia)*

2.2.2.6.2 Osteodysplasty (Melnick–Needles Syndrome)
2.2.2.6.3 Fuhrmann Dysplasia
2.2.2.6.4 Chromosomal Abnormalities

2.2.3 Vertebral Malsegmentation or Fusion

2.2.3.1 Malsegmentation

Malsegmentation of the spine (combinations of fused supernumerary, absent, and partially formed vertebrae) may be an isolated anomaly without diagnostic significance. It may also accompany neural tube defects or anorectal malformations. Malsegmentation is an important sign in several bone dysplasias, dysostoses, and syndromes and its presence necessitates a thorough clinical and radiographic appraisal. Imaging with CT and MR may be indicated.

Malsegmentation is a characteristic feature of the following:

2.2.3.1.1 Klippel–Feil Syndrome
2.2.3.1.2 Chondrodysplasia Punctata
2.2.3.1.3 Spondylocostal Dysostosis (Spondylothoracic Dysplasia)
2.2.3.1.4 Dyssegmental Dysplasia
2.2.3.1.5 Ateleosteogenesis Type II (de la Chapelle Dysplasia)
2.2.3.1.6 Robinow Type of Mesomelic Dysplasia
2.2.3.1.7 Myelomeningocele
2.2.3.1.8 Spondylocarpotarsal synostosis syndrome

Malsegmentation is a useful, but not diagnostic, sign in the following:

2.2.3.1.9 Cervico-oculo-acoustic Syndrome (Wildervanck Syndrome)
2.2.3.1.10 MURCS Association
2.2.3.1.11 Larsen Syndrome
2.2.3.1.12 Goltz Syndrome (Focal Dermal Hypoplasia)
2.2.3.1.13 Multiple Pterygium Syndrome
2.2.3.1.14 Aicardi Syndrome
2.2.3.1.15 Arteriohepatic Dysplasia
2.2.3.1.16 VATER (VACTERL) Association
2.2.3.1.17 Diastematomyelia
2.2.3.1.18 Split Notochord Syndrome
2.2.3.1.19 Chromosomal Abnormalities (Trisomy 18, Trisomy 8, Cri du Chat, etc.)
2.2.3.1.20 Foetal Alcohol Syndrome
2.2.3.1.21 Goldenhar Syndrome (Oculo-auriculo-vertebral Dysplasia)

2.2.3.1.22 Basal Cell Naevus Syndrome
2.2.3.1.23 Acrocephalosyndactylies

2.2.3.2   Fusion

2.2.3.2.1 Fusions of the Vertebral Bodies

Fusions of the vertebral bodies are of little importance in the radiographic recognition of bone dysplasias. Nevertheless, they occur in Klippel–Feil syndrome, spondylocostal dysostosis and as a frequent and important finding in the spondylocarpotarsal synostosis syndrome. Fusions of the vertebral bodies may represent sporadic congenital abnormalities, accompany chromosomal disorders, or result from infection or trauma. Anterior fusions may be a component of focal dermal hypoplasia (Goltz syndrome).

2.2.4   Vertebral Abnormalities – Miscellaneous

2.2.4.1   Coronal Clefts

Single coronal clefts may occasionally be seen in a normal vertebral column but they usually accompany severe bone dysostoses and dysplasias. They are often obliterated in the first few months of life but are sometimes observed later in childhood.

2.2.4.1.1   Malsegmentation of the Spine
2.2.4.1.2   Chondrodysplasia Punctata (Rhizomelic type)
2.2.4.1.3   Kniest Dysplasia
2.2.4.1.4   Metatropic Dysplasia
2.2.4.1.5   Fibrochondrogenesis
2.2.4.1.6   Dyssegmental Dysplasia
2.2.4.1.7   Atelosteogenesis (various forms)
2.2.4.1.8   Humerospinal Dysostosis
2.2.4.1.9   Taybi–Linder Syndrome (Cephaloskeletal Dysplasia)
2.2.4.1.10 Weissenbacher–Zweymüller Syndrome (Micrognathic Dwarfism)
2.2.4.1.11 Chromosomal Abnormalities (Trisomy 13)

2.2.4.2   Scalloping

Posterior scalloping of the vertebral bodies, usually of the lumbar spine, is an important sign in recognising narrowing of the spinal canal. It may occur either as an isolated anomaly (Congenital lumbar canal stenosis) or as a component of disorders that are usually accompanied by lumbar canal stenosis.

2.2.4.2.1 Achondroplasia
2.2.4.2.2 Hypochondroplasia
2.2.4.2.3 Dyggve–Melchior–Clausen Dysplasia
2.2.4.2.4 Smith–McCort Syndrome
2.2.4.2.5 Cockayne Syndrome
2.2.4.2.6 Cheirolumbar Dysostosis

Posterior scalloping of the vertebral bodies should be sought in patients suspected of having intraspinal tumours. It is an important sign in neurofibromatosis (due to dural ectasia, neurofibromata, or thoracic meningocele) and the rare distichiasis-lymphoedema syndrome (due to spinal extradural cysts).

Anterior scalloping of the vertebral bodies is of little importance in the recognition of bone dysplasias but it occurs in osteodysplasty (Melnick–Needles syndrome), Cockayne syndrome, and glycogen storage disease. It may also be a consequence of retroperitoneal or posterior mediastinal tumours or of aneurysms of the aorta.

2.2.4.3 Odontoid Hypoplasia

Hypoplasia of the odontoid process is a frequent finding in some bone dysplasias in which spinal involvement is severe. Although it is of little diagnostic value odontoid hypoplasia may cause instability of the suboccipital region especially if ligamentous laxity is also present (e.g. Down syndrome). In these circumstances instances of fatal atlanto-axial subluxation have been recorded.

2.2.4.3.1 Morquio Disease (MPS IV) and other Mucopolysaccharidoses
2.2.4.3.2 Mucolipidosis III
2.2.4.3.3 Spondylo-epiphyseal Dysplasias
2.2.4.3.4 "Classified" Spondylo-epi-metaphyseal Dysplasias such as Diastrophic Dysplasia, Metatropic Dysplasia
2.2.4.3.5 "Unclassified", Complex Spondylo-epi-metaphyseal Dysplasias
2.2.4.3.6 Dyggve–Melchior–Clausen Syndrome
2.2.4.3.7 Smith–McCort Syndrome
2.2.4.3.8 Isolated Hypoplasia of the Odontoid Process

2.2.4.4 Interpediculate Narrowing

Narrowing of the interpediculate distance on AP views of the lumbar spine rarely has clinical significance in childhood. However, this sign is useful in the recognition of some of the more common bone dysplasias, when shortening of the pedicles and narrowing of the canal will be evident on lateral projection. If there is unequivocal narrowing, long-term follow-up is indicated as damage to the spinal cord may occur later in life.

2.2.4.4.1   Hypochondroplasia
2.2.4.4.2   Achondroplasia
2.2.4.4.3   Thanatophoric Dysplasia
2.2.4.4.4   Diastrophic Dysplasia
2.2.4.4.5   Dyggve–Melchior–Clausen Syndrome
2.2.4.4.6   Smith–McCort Syndrome
2.2.4.4.7   Acrodysostosis
2.2.4.4.8   Pseudohypoparathyroidism and Pseudopseudohypoparathyroidism (Albright Hereditary Osteodystrophy)
2.2.4.4.9   Cheirolumbar Dysostosis
2.2.4.4.10 Hypophosphataemic Rickets
2.2.4.4.11 Turner Syndrome
2.2.4.4.12 Congenital Familial Lumbar Canal Stenosis
2.2.4.4.13 Chromosomal Abnormalities

2.2.4.5   Widening of the Spinal Canal

Widening of the spinal canal is a less useful sign than narrowing in the recognition of bone dysplasias. Widening is often accompanied by posterior scalloping of the vertebral bodies and it is an important finding in malformations of the spinal canal. In these circumstances further investigations such as CT, myelography or MR may be required

2.2.4.5.1   Neurofibromatosis (von Recklinghausen Disease)
2.2.4.5.2   Oto-palato-digital Syndrome
2.2.4.5.3   Myelomeningocele
2.2.4.5.4   Diastematomyelia
2.2.4.5.5   Distichiasis-Lymphoedema Syndrome

2.2.4.6   Sagittal Clefts (Butterfly vertebrae)

2.2.4.6.1   Aicardi Syndrome
2.2.4.6.2   Alagille Syndrome (Arteriohepatic Dysplasia)
2.2.4.6.3   Spondylothoracic Dysplasia

2.2.5   Calcification of the Intervertebral Discs

Calcification of the intervertebral discs is of little diagnostic value in the bone dysplasias. It is usually the result of degenerative changes of multifactorial aetiology, but it also occurs in a few genetic or congenital disorders.

2.2.5.1 Genetic or Congenital Disorders

2.2.5.1.1 Idiopathic
2.2.5.1.2 Congenital Spinal Fusion
2.2.5.1.3 Klippel–Feil Syndrome
2.2.5.1.4 Spondylo-epiphyseal Dysplasia Tarda
2.2.5.1.5 Homocystinuria
2.2.5.1.6 Alkaptonuria (Ochronosis)

2.2.5.2 Acquired Conditions

2.2.5.2.1 Juvenile Rheumatoid Arthritis
2.2.5.2.2 Ankylosing Spondylitis
2.2.5.2.3 Post-traumatic
2.2.5.2.4 Surgical Spinal Fusion
2.2.5.2.5 Degenerative
2.2.5.2.6 Gout
2.2.5.2.7 Pseudogout
2.2.5.2.8 Hyperparathyroidism
2.2.5.2.9 Hypervitaminosis D

2.3   Thorax

Rib anomalies are common in bone dysplasias and syndromic associations but they are rarely of diagnostic importance. Localised anomalies of one or two ribs are often seen in normal individuals. When more than two ribs are affected, a detailed search for other chest anomalies is obligatory. If several or all of the ribs are affected, skeletal survey is indicated.

Sternal anomalies although usually present in complex bone dysplasias are of little diagnostic value. Premature fusion of the sternal ossification centres is common in congenital heart disease. Associated chest deformities, notably pectus carinatum and excavatum can be better appreciated at clinical examination than on radiographs.

2.3.1   Rib Abnormalities

2.3.1.1	Short Ribs and Narrow Thorax
2.3.1.2	Absent Ribs
2.3.1.3	Supernumerary ribs
2.3.1.4	Narrow or Thin Ribs
2.3.1.5	Wide Ribs
2.3.1.6	Rib Malsegmentation
2.3.1.7	Rib Gaps
2.3.1.8	Cupped Ribs
2.3.1.9	Beaded Ribs

2.3.2   Clavicular Abnormalities

2.3.2.1	Congenital Clavicular Pseudoarthrosis
2.3.2.2	Skeletal Dysplasia
2.3.2.3	Skeletal Dysostosis
2.3.2.4	Miscellaneous Conditions
2.3.2.5	Clavicular Expansion
2.3.2.6	Hooked clavicles

2.3.3   Scapular Abnormalities

2.3.4   Glenoid Hypoplasia

2.3.5   Pectus Carinatum and Excavatum

2.3.1   Rib Abnormalities

2.3.1.1   Short Ribs and Narrow Thorax

A narrow thorax and short ribs are present in several bone dysplasias, many of which have a fatal outcome. In older children a long narrow thorax is the most important radiographic sign in asphyxiating thoracic dystrophy, Barnes syndrome (thoraco-pelvic dysostosis) and isolated thoracic dystrophy.

2.3.1.1.1   Achondrogenesis
2.3.1.1.2   Thanatophoric Dysplasia
2.3.1.1.3   Short Rib Syndromes
2.3.1.1.4   Asphyxiating Thoracic Dysplasia (Jeune Syndrome)
2.3.1.1.5   Chondroectodermal Dysplasia (Ellis–van Creveld Syndrome)
2.3.1.1.6   Metatropic Dysplasia
2.3.1.1.7   Achondroplasia
2.3.1.1.8   Hypophosphatasia
2.3.1.1.9   Barnes Syndrome (Thoraco-pelvic Dysostosis)
2.3.1.1.10 Isolated Thoracic Dysostosis

2.3.1.2   Absent Ribs

Absence of one or more ribs is an inconsistent feature of several bone dysplasias and syndromes, notably:

2.3.1.2.1   Campomelic Dysplasia
2.3.1.2.2   Cerebro-costo-mandibular Syndrome
2.3.1.2.3   Seckel Syndrome (Osteodysplastic, Primordial or Bird-headed Dwarfism)
2.3.1.2.4   Down Syndrome
2.3.1.2.5   Spondylocostal Dysostosis (Spondylothoracic Dysplasia)

2.3.1.3   Supernumerary Ribs

One or more additional ribs may represent an isolated developmental defect, especially in the cervical, lumbar, and sacrococcygeal regions. Supernumerary ribs are also a feature of the following:

2.3.1.3.1   VATER Association
2.3.1.3.2   Chromosomal Disorders (Trisomy 8, etc.)
2.3.1.3.3   Incontinentia Pigmenti

2.3.1.4   Narrow or Thin Ribs

Narrow ribs are present in many skeletal dysplasias. They may also be indicative of myopathy or hypotonia, and disorders of this type should be suspected if no additional bony abnormalities are present.

2.3.1.4.1   *Osteogenesis Imperfecta*
2.3.1.4.2   *Campomelic Dysplasia*
2.3.1.4.3   *Oculo-mandibulo-facial Syndrome (Hallermann–Streiff)*
2.3.1.4.4   *Achondrogenesis*
2.3.1.4.5   *Chondrodysplasia Punctata*
2.3.1.4.6   *Osteodysplasty (Melnick–Needles Syndrome)*
2.3.1.4.7   *Myopathies*
2.3.1.4.8   *Cockayne Syndrome*
2.3.1.4.9   *Neurofibromatosis (von Recklinghausen Disease)*
2.3.1.4.10 *Chromosomal Disorders (trisomy 13 and 18)*
2.3.1.4.11 *Skeletal Dysplasias with Gracile Bones*

2.3.1.5   Wide Ribs

The ribs are unduly wide in the following disorders:

2.3.1.5.1   *Complex Carbohydrate Metabolism Disorders (MPS and MLS)*
2.3.1.5.2   *Anaemias (notably Thalassaemia)*
2.3.1.5.3   *Metaphyseal Dysplasia (Pyle Disease)*
2.3.1.5.4   *Osteogenesis Imperfecta Congenita (Thick Bone Variety)*
2.3.1.5.5   *Lenz–Majewski Dysplasia*
2.3.1.5.6   *Myhre Syndrome*
2.3.1.5.7   *Trisomy 8*
2.3.1.5.8   *Schinzel–Giedion Syndrome*
2.3.1.5.9   *Cantu Syndrome*
2.3.1.5.10 *Craniometadiaphyseal Dysplasia, Wormian Bone Type*
2.3.1.5.11 *Craniometaphyseal Dysplasia*

2.3.1.6   Rib Malsegmentation

Minor rib malsegmentation in which bifid or fused ribs are present is a common finding on routine chest radiography. This is usually an isolated anomaly without clinical significance. However, if malsegmentation is more extensive and especially if it is accompanied by vertebral changes, it may be indicative of a bone dysplasia. In these circumstances further radiographic investigations should follow.

2.3.1.6.1   *Isolated Anomaly*

2.3.1.6.2   Spondylocostal Dysostosis (Spondylothoracic Dysplasia)
2.3.1.6.3   Focal Dermal Hypoplasia (Goltz Syndrome)
2.3.1.6.4   Naevoid Basal Cell Carcinoma Syndrome
2.3.1.6.5   Robinow Type of Mesomelic Dysplasia
2.3.1.6.6   Arteriohepatic Dysplasia
2.3.1.6.7   Diastematomyelia

2.3.1.7   Rib Gaps

Gaps due to radiolucent defects in the shafts of the ribs are an important diagnostic sign in the cerebro-costo-mandibular syndrome and Trisomy 8. They may occur in rare (or in some very rare) syndromic associations. The only other circumstance in which this appearance is produced is operative excision during cardiothoracic surgery.

2.3.1.8   Cupped Ribs

Anterior cupping of the ribs is common in chest radiographs of newborn premature infants. Rib cupping in a full-term infant or older child necessitates further radiological and biochemical investigations as it may be indicative of:

2.3.1.8.1   Bone Dysplasia, especially those with metaphyseal involvement – Metaphyseal Dysplasias, Spondylometaphyseal Dysplasias, and Narrow-Thorax Short-Rib Syndromes
2.3.1.8.2   Rickets (Dietary, Vitamin D-resistant Hypophosphataemic and Pseudo-vitamin D-deficient Rickets)
2.3.1.8.3   Rickets Secondary to Renal Disease, Anti-epileptic Drugs, Hepatic Disease, Tumours
2.3.1.8.4   Copper Metabolism Abnormalities (Infantile Nutritional Copper Deficiency; Menkes Kinky Hair Syndrome)

2.3.1.9   Beaded Ribs

2.3.1.9.1   Osteogenesis Imperfecta Type II
2.3.1.9.2   Achondrogenesis Type IA
2.3.1.9.3   Dappled Diaphyseal Dysplasia

2.3.2   Clavicular Abnormalities

Clavicular hypoplasia or dysplasia is a feature of a few skeletal disorders and multiple congenital anomaly syndromes (syndromic associations). It may also be present in conjunction with severe upper limb or spinal deficiencies.

2.3.2.1   Congenital Clavicular Pseudoarthrosis

Almost always on the right side. If on the left side, dextrocardia is usually present.

2.3.2.2   Skeletal Dysplasia

2.3.2.2.1   *Cleidocranial Dysplasia, classic autosomal dominant type*
2.3.2.2.2   *Cleidocranial Dysplasia, rare autosomal recessive type*
2.3.2.2.3   *Pycnodysostosis*

2.3.2.3   Skeletal Dysostosis

2.3.2.3.1   *Focal Dermal Hypoplasia (Goltz Syndrome)*
2.3.2.3.2   *Coffin–Siris Syndrome*

2.3.2.4   Miscellaneous Conditions

2.3.2.4.1   *Chromosomal Disorders (especially Trisomy 11, 13 and 18)*
2.3.2.4.2   *Primary Disturbances of Growth (notably Progeria)*
2.3.2.4.3   *Post-traumatic non-union*
2.3.2.4.4   *Restrictive Dermopathy*
2.3.2.4.5   *Yunis–Varon Syndrome*

2.3.2.5   Clavicular Expansion

Broad thickened clavicles are a common finding in osteosclerotic bone dysplasias, Caffey disease, multifocal recurrent osteomyelitis, and may be present in trisomy 8. Unilateral clavicular expansion occurs in histiocytosis X. The medial ends of the clavicles show gross expansion in oculo-dento-osseous dysplasia (rare autosomal recessive type), presenting a "mutton chop" configuration.

2.3.2.6   Hooked Clavicles

Hooked clavicles occur in several bone dysplasias and syndromic associations. As a diagnostic radiographic feature it is of secondary importance. These clavicular changes are usually accompanied by rib, vertebral and scapular abnormalities.

2.3.3 Scapular Abnormalities

Hypoplastic or small scapulae are important in the diagnosis of some bone dysplasias. This sign is easily missed if a systematic approach is not adopted.

2.3.3.1.1 *Cleidocranial Dysplasia*
2.3.3.1.2 *Osteo-onychodysplasia (Nail-patella Syndrome)*
2.3.3.1.3 *Achondrogenesis*
2.3.3.1.4 *Thanatophoric Dysplasia*
2.3.3.1.5 *Short-Rib Syndromes*
2.3.3.1.6 *Hypophosphatasia*
2.3.3.1.7 *Campomelic Dysplasia*
2.3.3.1.8 *Scapulo-iliac Dysplasia (Kosenow–Sinios Syndrome)*
2.3.3.1.9 *Atelosteogenesis II (La Chapelle Dysplasia)*
2.3.3.1.10 *Acampomelic Campomelic Dysplasia*
2.3.3.1.11 *Syndromic Associations – Various (e.g. Cumming Syndrome)*

2.3.4 Glenoid Hypoplasia

Glenoid hypoplasia is usually an isolated anomaly with dominant inheritance and variable penetrance. It is also a common finding in complex bone dysplasias such as spondyloepimetaphyseal dysplasias and in some syndromes. It is of secondary importance as a diagnostic radiographic sign of bone dysplasias.

2.3.5 Pectus Carinatum and Excavatum

Pectus carinatum and excavatum occur as isolated anomalies or as components of many bone dysplasias and syndromic associations. They can be better evaluated at clinically than by x-ray. As diagnostic radiographic findings these chest wall abnormalities are of secondary importance.

2.4   Pelvis

2.4.1   Pelvic Configuration

2.4.1.1   Short Sacro-iliac Notches
2.4.1.2   Crenated Iliac Crests
2.4.1.3   Retarded Pelvic Ossification
2.4.1.4   Narrow Pelvis
2.4.1.5   Unique Radiographic Features

2.4.2   Acetabular Abnormalities

2.4.2.1   Triradiate Acetabulum
2.4.2.2   Acetabular Protrusion

2.4.3   Femoral Head Abnormalities

2.4.3.1   Perthes Disease-like changes
2.4.3.2   Severely Delayed, Hypoplastic, or Absent Femoral Capital Epiphyses
2.4.3.3   Femoral Head Necrosis
2.4.3.4   Premature Ossification of the Femoral Capital Epiphyses

2.4.4   Femoral Neck Malalignment

2.4.4.1   Coxa Vara
2.4.4.2   Coxa Valga

2.4.5   Hip Dislocation

2.4.1   Pelvic Configuration

The pelvis has a characteristic configuration in several bone dysplasias. Although rarely specific, the presence of this feature limits the range of diagnostic possibilities. A normal pelvic radiogram, which includes the hips and lower lumbar spine, excludes the majority of the bone dysplasias.

2.4.1.1   Short Sacro-iliac Notches

2.4.1.1.1   Achondroplasia
2.4.1.1.2   Thanatophoric Dysplasia
2.4.1.1.3   Short Rib Syndrome Types I and III
2.4.1.1.4   Metatropic Dysplasia
2.4.1.1.5   Spondyloepimetaphyseal Dysplasias

2.4.1.2   Crenated Iliac Crests

2.4.1.2.1   Dyggve–Melchior–Clausen Dysplasia
2.4.1.2.2   Smith–McCort Syndrome
2.4.1.2.3   Parastremmatic Dysplasia
2.4.1.2.4   Enchondromatosis

2.4.1.3   Retarded Pelvic Ossification

2.4.1.3.1   Achondrogenesis Syndromes
2.4.1.3.2   Cleidocranial Dysplasia
2.4.1.3.3   Campomelic Dysplasia
2.4.1.3.4   Schinzel–Giedion Syndrome
2.4.1.3.5   Spondyloepimetaphyseal dysplasias

2.4.1.4   Narrow Pelvis

2.4.1.4.1   Campomelic Dysplasia
2.4.1.4.2   Osteodysplasty (Melnick–Needles Syndrome)
2.4.1.4.3   Acampomelic Campomelic Dysplasia

2.4.1.5   Unique Radiographic Features

2.4.1.5.1   Iliac Horns: osteo-onychodysplasia (Nail-patella Syndrome)
2.4.1.5.2   Ischio-pubic Gap: Patellar Hypoplasia Syndrome (Small Patella Syndrome)
2.4.1.5.3   Snail-shaped Ilia: Schneckenbecken Dysplasia
2.4.1.5.4   High Narrow Ilia: Campomelic Dysplasia
2.4.1.5.5   Gross Ilial Hypoplasia: Scapulo-iliac Dysplasia (Kosenow–Sinios Syndrome)
2.4.1.5.6   Small Iliac Angle: Down Syndrome

2.4.1.5.7   *Incomplete Ossification of the Ischial Rami –*
            Ischial-vertebral Dysplasia

2.4.2   Acetabular Abnormalities

2.4.2.1   Triradiate Acetabulum

The acetabulum has a triradiate configuration in infancy in the following
disorders:

2.4.2.1.1   *Achondroplasia*
2.4.2.1.2   *Chondroectodermal Dysplasia (Ellis–van Creveld*
            Syndrome)
2.4.2.1.3   *Asphyxiating Thoracic Dysplasia*
2.4.2.1.4   *Thanatophoric Dysplasia*

2.4.2.2   Acetabular Protrusion

Acetabular protrusion is a non-specific sign that is of little diagnostic value
in the bone dysplasias. If it is primary, it may be sporadic or familial.
Secondary acetabular protrusion occurs unilaterally in infection (acute
pyogenic, tuberculosis, traumatic) and bilaterally in the following:

2.4.2.2.1   *Metabolic Disorders*
2.4.2.2.2   *Degenerative Arthritis*
2.4.2.2.3   *Bone Dysplasia*

2.4.3   Femoral Head Abnormalities

2.4.3.1   Perthes Disease-like Changes

When ostensible bilateral Perthes disease is diagnosed, a generalised bone
dysplasia should be excluded. This differentiation is crucial, as untreated
Perthes disease may progress to femoral head necrosis. Changes of this
type may be present in the following:

2.4.3.1.1   *Spondylo-epiphyseal Dysplasia*
2.4.3.1.2   *Disorders of Complex Carbohydrate Metabolism (MPS*
            and MLS)
2.4.3.1.3   *Hypothyroidism*
2.4.3.1.4   *Meyer Dysplasia of the Femoral Capital Epiphyses*
2.4.3.1.5   *Trichorhinophalangeal Dysplasia Type I*
2.4.3.1.6   *Trichorhinophalangeal Dysplasia Type II (Giedion–*
            Langer)

2.4.3.1.7 Sickle Cell Disease
2.4.3.1.8 Spondylo-epi-metaphyseal Dysplasia
2.4.3.1.9 Geleophysic Dysplasia

2.4.3.2   Severely Delayed, Hypoplastic, or Absent Femoral Capital Epiphyses

2.4.3.2.1 Hypothyroidism
2.4.3.2.2 Spondylo-epiphyseal Dysplasia Congenita
2.4.3.2.3 Spondylo-epi-metaphyseal Dysplasia Congenita

2.4.3.3   Femoral Head Necrosis

Femoral head necrosis is usually "acquired", but it may also be a complication of the epiphyseal dysplasias. For this reason, if necrosis is bilateral, further investigations should be undertaken to exclude a generalised skeletal disorder.

2.4.3.3.1 Trauma and Microtrauma – Perthes Disease, Bone Dysplasias, Iatrogenic Necrosis of the Hip (during treatment of the opposite hip for dislocation), Femoral Neck Fracture.
2.4.3.3.2 Anaemias with Hyperplasia of the Marrow, notably Gaucher Disease
2.4.3.3.3 Sickle Cell Trait and Disease
2.4.3.3.4 Steroid Therapy
2.4.3.3.5 Acute and Chronic Pancreatitis (Fat Emboli or Enzymatic Damage of Vessels, as in Chronic Alcoholism)
2.4.3.3.6 Subacute Bacterial Endocarditis
2.4.3.3.7 Nitrogen Emboli
2.4.3.3.8 Hypertension
2.4.3.3.9 Arteriosclerosis
2.4.3.3.10 Gout

2.4.3.4   Premature Ossification of the Femoral Capital Epiphyses

2.4.3.4.1 Chondroectodermal Dysplasia (Ellis–van Creveld Syndrome)
2.4.3.4.2 Asphyxiating Thoracic Dysplasia (Jeune Syndrome)
2.4.3.4.3 Short Rib Syndrome Type I (Saldino–Noonan Syndrome)

2.4.4   Femoral Neck Malalignment

2.4.4.1   Coxa Vara

Coxa vara is a common non-specific finding in many different, unrelated bone diseases. Absence of this malalignment virtually excludes some bone dysplasias. Conversely, its presence necessitates further investigation, especially if there is bilateral involvement.

2.4.4.1.1   *Spondylo-epiphyseal Dysplasia Congenita*
2.4.4.1.2   *Spondylometaphyseal Dysplasia (Kozlowski Type)*
2.4.4.1.3   *Spondylo-epi-metaphyseal Dysplasia (various types)*
2.4.4.1.4   *Spondylometaphyseal Dysplasia (Sutcliffe or Corner Fracture Type)*
2.4.4.1.5   *Spondylometaphyseal Dysplasia (Algerian Type)*
2.4.4.1.6   *Metaphyseal Chondrodysplasias (notably Schmid Type)*
2.4.4.1.7   *Frontometaphyseal Dysplasia*
2.4.4.1.8   *Cleidocranial Dysplasia*
2.4.4.1.9   *Osteodysplasty (Melnick–Needles Syndrome)*
2.4.4.1.10   *Dyggve–Melchior–Clausen Syndrome*
2.4.4.1.11   *Smith–McCort Syndrome*
2.4.4.1.12   *Coffin–Lowry Syndrome*
2.4.4.1.13   *Femoral Facial Syndrome (Proximal Focal Femoral Dysplasia)*
2.4.4.1.14   *Fibrous Dysplasia*
2.4.4.1.15   *Idiopathic Coxa Vara*
2.4.4.1.16   *Post-traumatic Coxa Vara*

2.4.4.2   Coxa Valga

Coxa valga is a common non-specific finding in many different conditions. However, its presence has diagnostic significance in syndromes of muscular hypotonia and in complex carbohydrate disorders (MPS and MLS).

2.4.5   Hip Dislocation

Hip dislocation or subluxation is a non-specific finding that may occur as an isolated anomaly or as part of many different syndromes. In bilateral CDH, an underlying bone dysplasia must be excluded. When multiple joint dislocations are present, the genetic hypermobility syndromes should be suspected (see Section 1).

2.5   Long Bones

2.5.1   Alterations in Density

2.5.2   Alterations in Contours

2.5.3   Limb Shortening

2.5.4   Abnormalities of the Long Bones of the Forearms

2.5.5   Abnormalities of the Long Bones of the Legs

2.5.6   Epiphyseal Abnormalities

2.5.7   Metaphyseal Abnormalities

2.5.7.1   Metaphyseal Chondrodysplasias
2.5.7.2   Metabolic Disorders

2.5.8   Diaphyseal Abnormalities

2.5.8.1   Medullary Stenosis
2.5.8.2   Gracile Slender Long Bones

2.5.1 Alterations in Density

The density of the long bones is increased or decreased in a number of generalised skeletal disorders that are listed in Section 1. Linear striations, which are a sclerotic anomaly of trabecular pattern, are present in the long bones in several bone dysplasias and syndromes.

2.5.1.1 Linear Striations

2.5.1.1.1 *Osteopathia Striata*
2.5.1.1.2 *Osteopathia Striata with Craniosclerosis*
2.5.1.1.3 *Osteopoikilosis*
2.5.1.1.4 *Melorheostosis*
2.5.1.1.5 *Enchondromatosis (Ollier Disease)*
2.5.1.1.6 *Osteopetrosis*
2.5.1.1.7 *Polyostotic Fibrous Dysplasia*
2.5.1.1.8 *Neurofibromatosis (von Recklinghausen Disease)*
2.5.1.1.9 *Goltz Syndrome (Focal Dermal Hypoplasia)*
2.5.1.1.10 *Aarskog Syndrome*

2.5.1.2 Transverse Bands of Increased Density

Transverse bands of increased density are a frequent finding in osteopetrosis. Narrow and denser "arrested growth lines" are often encountered in normal individuals, and testify to previous non-specific disease. They may also be an expression of a continuing metabolic disorder or infection.

2.5.1.2.1 *Osteopetrosis (all forms)*
2.5.1.2.2 *"Arrested Growth" Lines*
2.5.1.2.3 *Neoplasia (Leukaemia, Neuroblastoma)*

2.5.1.3 Transverse Bands of Decreased Density

Transverse bands of decreased density have limited diagnostic value. They are usually present in osteopetrosis and are often seen in normal neonates. They may be a sign of a metabolic disease or of neoplastic conditions such as leukaemia and neuroblastoma.

2.5.1.3.1 *Osteopetrosis (all forms)*
2.5.1.3.2 *Metabolic Disorders*
2.5.1.3.3 *Neoplasia (Leukaemia, Neuroblastoma)*

2.5.2 Alterations in Contours

2.5.2.1 Non-specific Predominantly Diaphyseal Widening

Increased diameter or widening of the long bones is a common and important sign in many conditions, including metabolic disorders, bone dysplasias, and blood diseases. Widening of the long bones may also be produced by periosteal thickening consequent upon chronic periostitis (see Section 1). Increased diameter of the bones, especially the diaphyses, occurs in the following:

2.5.2.1.1 *Cranio-diaphyseal Dysplasia (ribs, clavicles, diaphyses)*

2.5.2.1.2 *Osteoectasia with Hyperphosphatasia (tubular bones, skull)*

2.5.2.1.3 *Oculo-dento-osseous Dysplasia (tubular bones, ribs, clavicles)*

2.5.2.1.4 *Endosteal Hyperostosis (van Buchem Disease)*

2.5.2.1.5 *Pachydermoperiostosis (Idiopathic Hypertrophic Osteoarthropathy)*

2.5.2.1.6 *Infantile Cortical Hyperostosis (Caffey Disease)*

2.5.2.1.7 *Singleton–Merten Syndrome*

2.5.2.1.8 *Dysosteosclerosis*

2.5.2.1.9 *Osteopetrosis*

2.5.2.1.10 *Diaphyseal Dysplasia (Camurati–Engelmann Disease)*

2.5.2.1.11 *Fibrous Dysplasia*

2.5.2.1.12 *Neurofibromatosis (von Recklinghausen Disease) [subperiosteal haemorrhages]*

2.5.2.1.13 *Complex Carbohydrate Metabolism Disorders (MPS and MLS)*

2.5.2.1.14 *Lipid Storage Disorders*

2.5.2.1.15 *Infections (Tuberculosis)*

2.5.2.1.16 *Trisomy 8 (ribs)*

2.5.2.1.17 *Tumours (Neuroblastoma)*

2.5.2.2 Metaphyseal Widening

Broad metaphyses are usually a sign of severe bone disease. Minor widening is present in numerous metabolic disorders and many different syndromes, but these borderline changes are usually without diagnostic significance. The conditions in which metaphyseal widening is an important feature are listed below:

2.5.2.2.1 *Metaphyseal Dysplasia (Pyle Disease)*

2.5.2.2.2 *Frontometaphyseal Dysplasia*

2.5.3   Limb Shortening

Limb shortening is categorised as follows:

Rhizomelia:	proximal shortening involving the humerus or femur
Mesomelia:	shortening of the mid-portions of the limbs, involving the forearms (radius and ulna) and the lower legs (tibia and fibula)
Acromelia:	shortening of the bones of the hands and feet (see 2.6)

Combinations of these types of limb shortening often occur but categorisation of the patient in terms of the changes that predominate is of diagnostic value.

2.5.3.1   Rhizomelic (Proximal) Limb Shortening

The syndromes in which there is predominant rhizomelic shortening are listed below. Some rhizomelia is present in most bone dysplasias that are associated with short stature and mesomelic shortening of the extremities.

2.5.3.1.7   *Femoral Facial Syndrome (Proximal Focal Femoral Dysplasia)*
2.5.3.1.8   *Trauma (Battered Child)*

2.5.3.2   Mesomelic (Mid-portion) Limb Shortening

Mesomelic dysplasias are a heterogeneous group of more than 30 disorders characterised by disproportionate shortening of the middle segment of the extremities. These skeletal dysplasias can be subcategorised by the presence or absence of involvement of the hands and feet. Radiographic studies are often of great importance in the mesomelia syndromes as characteristic features that permit diagnostic precision may be present. The mesomelic dysplasias listed below show specific radiographic features. Dyschondrosteosis is more common than the total of all other mesomelic dysplasias.

Mesomelia with normal hands and feet:

2.5.3.2.1   *Dyschondrosteosis*
2.5.3.2.2   *Mesomelic Dysplasia (Langer Type)*
2.5.3.2.3   *Mesomelic Dysplasia with Relative Shortening of the Fibulae (Rheinhardt–Pfeiffer Type)*
2.5.3.2.4   *Mesomelic Dysplasia with Elongation of Fibulae*
2.5.3.2.5   *Kozlowski–Reardon Type*

Mesomelia with hand and foot abnormalities:

2.5.3.2.6   *Acromesomelic Dysplasias*
2.5.3.2.7   *Mesomelic Dysplasia (Nievergelt Type)*
2.5.3.2.8   *Mesomelic Dysplasia (Robinow Type)*
2.5.3.2.9   *Mesomelic Dysplasia (Werner Type)*
2.5.3.2.10 *Mesomelic Dysplasia (Hypoplastic Tibia and Radius Type)*
2.5.3.2.11 *Grebe Dysplasia*

2.5.4   Abnormalities of the Long Bones of the Forearms

2.5.4.1   Radio-ulnar Synostosis

Radio-ulnar synostosis may occur sporadically, in isolation and as an autosomal dominant trait. It is often associated with radial head dislocation and synostosis of one or more cranial sutures, sometimes at random with anomalies of the hands and lower extremities. In addition, bony bridges form in Caffey disease and in fibrodysplasia ossificans progressiva, while the interosseous ligaments can ossify following trauma in osteogenesis imperfecta. Radio-ulnar synostosis is a common feature in the conditions listed below:

2.5.4.1.1 *Multiple Cartilaginous Exostoses (distal forearm)*
2.5.4.1.2 *Multiple Synostoses (see Carpal and Tarsal Fusion, 2.6.3.1)*
2.5.4.1.3 *Mesomelic Dysplasia (Nievergelt Type)*
2.5.4.1.4 *Holt–Oram Syndrome*
2.5.4.1.5 *Acrocephalosyndactyly*
2.5.4.1.6 *Klinefelter and Other Cytogenetic Syndromes with Supernumerary X Chromosomes*
2.5.4.1.7 *Foetal Alcohol Syndrome*
2.5.4.1.8 *Thalidomide Embryopathy*
2.5.4.1.9 *Antley–Bixler Syndrome (more often radio-humeral synostosis)*

2.5.4.2 Madelung Deformity

The Madelung deformity is usually sporadic and it may be unilateral or bilateral. If it is bilateral, the diagnostic possibility of dyschondrosteosis always warrants consideration.

2.5.4.2.1 *Dyschondrosteosis*
2.5.4.2.2 *Multiple Cartilaginous Exostoses (Diaphyseal Aclasis)*
2.5.4.2.3 *Turner Syndrome*
2.5.4.2.4 *Trauma*
2.5.4.2.5 *Infection*

2.5.4.3 Radial Hypoplasia-aplasia

Defects of the radial ray and associated anomalies comprise a heterogeneous group of disorders. Radial hypoplasia is an important sign in the mesomelic dysplasias and other well-defined syndromes. It is often associated with multisystem abnormalities including cutaneous, skeletal, haematological, cardiac, renal and craniofacial anomalies. Radial hypoplasia is of diagnostic importance in the following:

2.5.4.3.1 *Fanconi Anaemia*
2.5.4.3.2 *Thrombocytopenia-Absent Radius (TAR) Syndrome*
2.5.4.3.3 *Craniosynostoses (some forms, such as the Baller–Gerold Syndrome)*
2.5.4.3.4 *Cornelia de Lange Syndrome*
2.5.4.3.5 *VATER Association*
2.5.4.3.6 *Mesomelic Dysplasias (See Mesomelic Limb Shortening)*
2.5.4.3.7 *Radial Ray Reduction Syndromes (Holt–Oram, RAPADILINO, Roberts, and Pseudothalidomide Syndromes)*

2.5.4.3.8   *Phocomelia*
2.5.4.3.9   *Treacher Collins Syndrome (Mandibulofacial*
dysostosis)
2.5.4.3.10   *Seckel Syndrome*
2.5.4.3.11   *Atelosteogenesis II (de la Chapelle Dysplasia)*
2.5.4.3.12   *Rothmund–Thomson Syndrome*
2.5.4.3.13   *Chromosome Abnormalities (Trisomy 13, 18)*

2.5.4.4   Ulnar Hypoplasia-aplasia

Defects in the ulnar rays often accompany radial ray defects, hand defects and other bony abnormalities. Ulnar hypoplasia-aplasia is of diagnostic importance in:

2.5.4.4.1   *Mesomelic Dysplasias*
2.5.4.4.2   *Acro-mesomelic Dysplasias*
2.5.4.4.3   *Cornelia de Lange Syndrome*
2.5.4.4.4   *Femur-fibula-ulnar Syndrome*
2.5.4.4.5   *Weyers Oligodactyly Syndrome*
2.5.4.4.6   *Ulnar Defect with Symphalangism*

2.5.4.5   Elbow Joint or Radial Head Hypoplasia with Dislocation or Subluxation

Elbow joint subluxation or dislocation may be an isolated anomaly but more often it is a component of a specific skeletal dysplasia syndrome. Dislocations of this type also occur in the articular hypermobility syndromes (see Section 1).

2.5.4.5.1   *Osteo-onychodysplasia (Nail-patella Syndrome)*
2.5.4.5.2   *Multiple Synostoses Syndrome*
2.5.4.5.3   *Oto-palato-digital Syndrome*
2.5.4.5.4   *Craniofacial Dysostosis*
2.5.4.5.5   *Mesomelic Dysplasia (Nievergelt Type)*
2.5.4.5.6   *Seckel Syndrome*
2.5.4.5.7   *Coffin–Siris Syndrome*
2.5.4.5.8   *Cornelia de Lange Syndrome*
2.5.4.5.9   *Spondylo-epi-metaphyseal Dysplasia with Joint Laxity*
2.5.4.5.10   *Humerospinal Dysostosis*
2.5.4.5.11   *Omodysplasia*
2.5.4.5.12   *Chromosomal Abnormalities (Klinefelter and other*
Supernumerary X Syndromes)

2.5.5   Abnormalities of the Long Bones of the Legs

2.5.5.1   Bowed Legs and Genu Varum

Bowing of the legs is usually a result of deformity of the shafts of the tibia and fibula. It may also be the consequence of genu varum and often both abnormalities are present in varying degrees. Extreme bowing of the femora is characteristic of the Fuhrmann syndrome. Physiological bowing of infancy is by far the most common form of bowlegs.

> *2.5.5.1.1   Achondroplasia*
> *2.5.5.1.2   Pseudochondroplasia*
> *2.5.5.1.3   Hypochondroplasia*
> *2.5.5.1.4   Metaphyseal Chondrodysplasias (especially Schmid Type)*
> *2.5.5.1.5   Spondylometaphyseal Dysplasias (heterogeneous)*
> *2.5.5.1.6   Spondylo-epi-metaphyseal Dysplasias (heterogeneous)*
> *2.5.5.1.7   Boomerang Dysplasia*
> *2.5.5.1.8   Kyphomelic Dysplasia*
> *2.5.5.1.9   Blount Disease*
> *2.5.5.1.10 Hypophosphataemia (Vitamin D-resistant rickets)*
> *2.5.5.1.11 Campomelic Dysplasia*

2.5.5.2   Genu Valgum

> *2.5.5.2.1   MPS IV (Morquio Disease)*
> *2.5.5.2.2   Spondylo-epiphyseal Dysplasia (some forms)*
> *2.5.5.2.3   Spondylometaphyseal Dysplasia (some forms)*
> *2.5.5.2.4   Spondylometaphyseal Dysplasia (Schmidt and Algerian Types)*

2.5.5.3   Isolated Tibial Bowing

Isolated congenital tibial bowing is a rare anomaly. If it is accompanied by pseudoarthrosis the diagnosis should be regarded as neurofibromatosis until proved otherwise. Reverse tibial bowing is a characteristic sign of SADDAN dysplasia.

> *2.5.5.3.1   Neurofibromatosis (von Recklinghausen Disease) [usually lateral bowing]*
> *2.5.5.3.2   Osteofibrous Dysplasia of the Tibia and Fibula (Campanacci Syndrome)*
> *2.5.5.3.3   Absence or Hypoplasia of Fibula*
> *2.5.5.3.4   SADDAN Dysplasia*
> *2.5.5.3.5   Idiopathic Anterior or Posterior Tibial Bowing*
> *2.5.5.3.6   Trauma*
> *2.5.5.3.7   Osteitis*

2.5.5.4   Patellar Hypoplasia

Hypoplasia or dysplasia of the patella is an important radiographic sign in osteo-onychodysplasia. It may be present in some types of spondylo-epiphyseal dysplasia, as well as in other conditions as listed below:

2.5.5.4.1   *Osteo-onychodysplasia (Nail-patella syndrome)*
2.5.5.4.2   *Spondylo-epiphyseal Dysplasia (Heterogeneous)*
2.5.5.4.3   *Spondylo-epi-metaphyseal Dysplasia (Heterogeneous)*
2.5.5.4.4   *Patellar Hypoplasia Syndrome (Small Patella Syndrome)*
2.5.5.4.5   *RAPADILINO Syndrome*
2.5.5.4.6   *Arthrogryposis Syndromes*
2.5.5.4.7   *Mesomelic Dysplasia (Werner type)*
2.5.5.4.8   *Mesomelic Dysplasia (Hypoplastic Tibia and Radius type)*
2.5.5.4.9   *Trisomy 8*

2.5.5.5   Elongation of Fibula

Apparent elongation of the fibula is usually relative to shortening of the tibia. Although without great diagnostic significance, proximal or distal fibular elongation is sometimes an obvious sign that deserves consideration. It is the most characteristic bony sign in the serpentine fibula-polycystic kidney syndrome.

2.5.5.5.1   *Achondroplasia*
2.5.5.5.2   *Hypochondroplasia*
2.5.5.5.3   *Pseudoachondroplasia*
2.5.5.5.4   *Metaphyseal Chondrodysplasia (McKusick type)*
2.5.5.5.5   *Mesomelic Dysplasia (some forms)*
2.5.5.5.6   *Spondylo-epi-metaphyseal Dysplasias (Ill-defined types)*
2.5.5.5.7   *Serpentine Fibula-Polycystic Kidney Syndrome*
2.5.5.5.8   *Myopathies*

2.5.5.6   Fibular Hypoplasia

Fibular hypoplasia usually accompanies hypoplasia of the tibia. Predominance of the changes in the fibula is sometimes a useful sign in the following dysplasias:

2.5.5.6.1   *Campomelic Dysplasia*
2.5.5.6.2   *Chondroectodermal Dysplasia (Ellis–van Creveld Syndrome)*
2.5.5.6.3   *Atelosteogenesis II (La Chapelle Dysplasia)*
2.5.5.6.4   *Seckel Syndrome*
2.5.5.6.5   *Chromosomal Abnormalities*

2.5.6   Epiphyseal abnormalities

2.5.6.1   Stippled Epiphyses

Irregularities of enchondral ossification of the epiphyses produces an appearance of multiple small radio-opaque spots or "stippling". These changes are sometimes accompanied by involvement of the metaphyses and spine. The unequivocal presence of stippled or punctate epiphyses significantly narrows the diagnostic possibilities, but it must be emphasised that minor stippling can be a normal variant. Stippling is always transient and disappears after infancy.

2.5.6.1.1   *Chondrodysplasia Punctata (Rhizomelic, Dominant and X-linked forms)*
2.5.6.1.2   *Warfarin Embryopathy*
2.5.6.1.3   *Foetal Alcohol Syndrome*
2.5.6.1.4   *Zellweger Syndrome (Cerebro-hepato-renal Syndrome) [patellar stippling]*
2.5.6.1.5   *Smith–Lemli–Opitz Syndrome*
2.5.6.1.6   *GMI Gangliosidosis*
2.5.6.1.7   *De Barsy Syndrome*
2.5.6.1.8   *Chromosomal Abnormalities (Down Syndrome, Trisomy 18 and others)*
2.5.6.1.9   *Hypothyroidism*
2.5.6.1.10 *Infection (Listeria monocytogenes)*
2.5.6.1.11 *Spondyloepimetaphyseal Dysplasia, Short Limb, Abnormal Calcification type*

2.5.6.2   Epiphyseal Hypoplasia, Dysplasia, or Dysgenesis

Epiphyseal hypoplasia, dysplasia, or dysgenesis is a common finding in many bone dysplasias. However, the diagnosis is complicated by the fact that borderline or minor epiphyseal changes are present in virtually every skeletal dysplasia syndrome and in metabolic disorders, dysostoses, chromosomal conditions, and malformations. For the sake of diagnostic clarity, it is therefore sometimes easier to disregard minimal epiphyseal abnormalities.

2.5.6.2.1   *Hypothyroidism*
2.5.6.2.2   *Perthes Disease*
2.5.6.2.3   *Meyer Dysplasia (femoral capital epiphyses)*
2.5.6.2.4   *Multiple Epiphyseal Dysplasia (heterogeneous)*
2.5.6.2.5   *Spondylo-epiphyseal Dysplasia Congenita*
2.5.6.2.6   *Spondylo-epiphyseal Dysplasia Tarda*
2.5.6.2.7   *Spondylo-epi-metaphyseal dysplasia (heterogeneous)*

2.5.6.2.8   *Arthro-ophthalmopathy (Stickler syndrome)*
2.5.6.2.9   *Osteo-onychodysplasia (Nail-patella Syndrome)*
2.5.6.2.10 *Trichorhinophalangeal Syndromes I and II*
2.5.6.2.11 *Metatropic Dysplasia*
2.5.6.2.12 *Kniest Dysplasia*
2.5.6.2.13 *Pseudoachondroplasia*
2.5.6.2.14 *Diastrophic Dysplasia*
2.5.6.2.15 *Pseudodiastrophic Dysplasia*
2.5.6.2.16 *Parastremmatic Dysplasia*
2.5.6.2.17 *Dyggve–Melchior–Clausen Dysplasia*
2.5.6.2.18 *Smith–McCort Syndrome*
2.5.6.2.19 *Walcott–Rallison Syndrome*

2.5.6.3   Cone-shaped Epiphyses of Long Bones

Cone-shaped epiphyses of the small tubular bones are common and are sometimes an important diagnostic sign. Those of the long tubular bones are much rarer but of great diagnostic value. They occur in:

2.5.6.3.1   *Acroscyphodysplasia (various types)*
2.5.6.3.2   *Osteoglophonic Dysplasia*
2.5.6.3.3   *Multiple Metaphyseal Osteomyelitis*
2.5.6.3.4   *Hypervitaminosis A*
2.5.6.3.5   *Trauma*

2.5.6.4   Large Epiphyses of Long Bones

Large epiphyses occur in cleidocranial dysplasia and they are also a prominent feature of several very rare bone dysplasias:

2.5.6.4.1   *Oto-spondylo-megaepiphyseal Dysplasia (OSMED)*
2.5.6.4.2   *Spondylo-megaepiphyseal Metaphyseal Dysplasia*
2.5.6.4.3   *Progressive Pseudorheumatoid Dysplasia*
2.5.6.4.4   *Macroepiphyseal Dysplasia with Osteoporosis*
2.5.6.4.5   *Short Syndrome*
2.5.6.4.6   *Neonatal Syndrome of Multisystem Inflammation*

2.5.7   Metaphyseal Abnormalities

Metaphyseal irregularity, cupping or widening is present in dietary and metabolic rickets and in several bone dysplasias. In the former conditions the skeleton may be osteoporotic, while in the latter disorders abnormalities in regions other than the metaphyses are usually present. Minimal or borderline metaphyseal changes may be seen in many other metabolic disorders, and malformation syndromes, but in these situations the abnormality is of little diagnostic significance. Metaphyseal anomalies are also a component of the spondylo-epi-metaphyseal dysplasias and related disorders in which spinal changes predominate, and which have been listed in Section 2.2.

2.5.7.1 Metaphyseal Chondrodysplasias

2.5.7.1.1 Jansen Type
2.5.7.1.2 Schmid Type
2.5.7.1.3 McKusick Type (Cartilage Hair Hypoplasia)
2.5.7.1.4 Schwachman Type (with Pancreatic Insufficiency and Bone Marrow Dysfunction)
2.5.7.1.5 Metaphyseal Dysplasia Spahr Type
2.5.7.1.6 Metaphyseal Anadysplasia (regressive metaphyseal dysplasia)
2.5.7.1.7 Acroscyphodysplasia (various types)
2.5.7.1.8 Adenosine Deaminase deficiency
2.5.7.1.9 Other Types

2.5.7.2 Metabolic Disorders

2.5.7.2.1 Dietary Rickets
2.5.7.2.2 Hypophosphataemia
2.5.7.2.3 Renal and Other Forms of Metabolic Rickets
2.5.7.2.4 Infantile Nutritional Copper Deficiency
2.5.7.2.5 Menkes Kinky Hair Syndrome
2.5.7.2.6 Adenosine Deaminase Deficiency

Similar metaphyseal changes can be observed after trauma or infection and in scurvy, sickle cell anaemia, hypervitaminosis A, and homocystinuria. Desferoxamine, used in the treatment of thalassaemia major, may induce similar bony changes.

2.5.8 Diaphyseal Abnormalities

2.5.8.1 Medullary Stenosis

2.5.8.1.1 Kenny–Caffey Syndrome
2.5.8.1.2 Melnick–Needles Syndrome
2.5.8.1.3 Pycnodysostosis
2.5.8.1.4 Endosteal Hyperostosis (Worth, van Buchem, Nakamura)

2.5.8.2 Gracile (Slender Long Bones)

2.5.8.2.1 Gracile Bone Dysplasias (various forms)

2.6   Hands and Feet

Radiological examination of the hands and feet, including the wrists and ankles, often provides important diagnostic clues. It is self-evident that study of the hands is likely to be diagnostically more productive than study of the feet, but the feet should never be neglected.

Abnormalities are listed in this chapter in the order in which they would generally be appraised by the radiologist, and they range from generalised changes of bone length and texture to localised anomalies at specific sites. Radiographic signs that are of little value in recognition of bone dysplasias are omitted from this account.

Well-defined developmental abnormalities such as syndactyly, polydactyly, and symphalangism may occur in isolation or as components of numerous syndromes. The value of clinical examination greatly exceeds that of radiographic investigation of digital anomalies of this type, and for this reason they also have been excluded from this chapter.

2.6.1   Shortening of the Hands and Feet

2.6.1.1   Generalised Shortening
2.6.1.2   Metacarpal Shortening

2.6.2   Epiphyseal Abnormalities in the Hands and Feet

2.6.2.1   Cone-Shaped epiphyses
2.6.2.2   Pseudoepiphyses
2.6.2.3   Dense Sclerotic Epiphyses

2.6.3   Carpus and Tarsus

2.6.3.1   Fusions
2.6.3.2   Supernumerary Ossification Centres

2.6.4   Thumb Abnormalities

2.6.4.1   Thumb Hypoplasia, Aplasia, or Agenesis
2.6.4.2   Finger-like or Triphalangeal Thumb

2.6.5   Acro-osteolysis

2.6.5.1   Idiopathic Osteolysis, Predominantly Phalangeal
2.6.5.2   Idiopathic Osteolysis, Predominantly Carpo-tarsal
2.6.5.3   Acro-osteolysis with Neurological Deficit
2.6.5.4   Acro-osteolysis without Neurological Deficit

2.6.1   Shortening of the Hands and Feet

2.6.1.1   Generalised Shortening

Generalised shortening of the hands and feet (acromelia) is infrequently found in isolation; more often other regions of the body are also affected. Although the shortening is clinically obvious, radiographs give insight into the precise nature of the skeletal abnormalities. Acromelia has practical significance in that its absence or presence permits diagnostic exclusion of several bone dysplasias. Pattern profile analysis by the method of Poznanski, in which relative lengths of the tubular bones are expressed graphically in terms of their standard deviations from the norm, is a valuable technique for objective appraisal of acromelia.

Digital shortening can be generalised or limited to the distal, middle or proximal phalanges, little finger or thumb. Brachydactyly is often associated with cone shaped epiphyses, sometimes with polydactyly or syndactyly.

In many bone dysplasias, the most important changes are in the hands. Other bones can be affected but the abnormalities are usually less characteristic and inconstant. In some of them hand abnormalities are discreet and can be easily overlooked (e.g. acromicric and geleophysic dysplasia). At the other end of the spectrum are bone dysplasias with distinctive bony changes in the hands. (e.g. trichorhinophalangeal syndrome, angel-shaped phalango-epiphyseal dysplasia (ASPED) and brachydactyly syndromes). Normal hand radiographs exclude all of these latter disorders.

Other hand and foot anomalies like split hand and foot, syndactyly, claw hand, large hand, large broad thumb and big toe are better appreciated at clinical examination than on X-ray. Although they occur sporadically in bone dysplasias, their presence is essential for the diagnosis of several syndromic associations. In bone dysplasias they are overshadowed by other, more important characteristic findings.

Digital shortening is a feature of the following conditions:

2.6.1.1.1   *Achondroplasia*
2.6.1.1.2   *Pseudoachondroplasia*
2.6.1.1.3   *Acrodysostosis and other "Peripheral Dysostoses"*
2.6.1.1.4   *Acromesomelic Dysplasia (Maroteaux type)*
2.6.1.1.5   *Acromesomelic Dysplasia (Campailla–Martinelli type)*
2.6.1.1.6   *Disorders of Complex Carbohydrate Metabolism (MPS and MLS)*
2.6.1.1.7   *Spondylo-epi-metaphyseal Dysplasia (heterogeneous)*
2.6.1.1.8   *Pseudohypoparathyroidism (Albright Hereditary Osteodystrophy)*
2.6.1.1.9   *Acromicric Dysplasia*
2.6.1.1.10 *Geleophysic Dysplasia*

2.6.1.1.11 *Neonatal Short-limb Dysplasias, notably*
               Thanatophoric Dysplasia
2.6.1.1.12 *Binder Syndrome (Maxillonasal Dysplasia)*
2.6.1.1.13 *EEC Syndrome (Adams–Oliver Syndrome)*
2.6.1.1.14 *Grebe Dysplasia*
2.6.1.1.15 *Angel-shaped Phalango Epiphyseal Dysplasia (ASPED)*
2.6.1.1.16 *Weill-Marchesani Syndrome*
2.6.1.1.17 *Cranioectodermal Dysplasia*
2.6.1.1.18 *Punctate Epiphyseal Dysplasia (various forms)*

2.6.1.2 Metacarpal Shortening

Isolated shortening of the fourth metacarpal is a non-specific finding in many bone dysplasias; it also occurs in isolation and as a component of the Turner syndrome and of pseudohypoparathyroidism. Non-specific, isolated, or syndromic shortening of the other metacarpals, especially the third and fifth, is also fairly common. Shortening of the metacarpals is frequent in the following conditions:

2.6.1.2.1 *Brachydactyly Syndromes*
2.6.1.2.2 *Turner Syndrome*
2.6.1.2.3 *Pseudohypoparathyroidsm*
2.6.1.2.4 *Basal Cell Naevus Carcinoma Syndrome*
2.6.1.2.5 *Trichorhinophalangeal Syndrome Type I*
2.6.1.2.6 *Beckwith–Wiedemann Syndrome*
2.6.1.2.7 *Russell–Silver Syndrome*
2.6.1.2.8 *Marinesco–Sjogren Syndrome*
2.6.1.2.9 *Chromosomal Disorders*

2.6.2 Epiphyseal Abnormalities

2.6.2.1 Cone-shaped Epiphyses

Cone-shaped epiphyses are an important diagnostic sign in numerous bone dysplasias and they are common in many syndromic associations. Equally, their absence virtually rules out many entities. They may also occur as a normal variant, especially in the toes, following trauma and infection, and in hypervitaminosis A.

Cone-shaped epiphyses are a significant feature of the following conditions:

2.6.2.1.1 *Acrodysostosis*
2.6.2.1.2 *Trichorhinophalangeal Dysplasia Types I and II*
2.6.2.1.3 *Asphyxiating Thoracic Dysplasia*

2.6.2.2   Pseudoepiphyses

Transverse notching at the base of the second and fifth metacarpals is a common variant that is present in about 30% of normal persons. Significant notching and pseudoepiphyses are fairly common in ill-defined mental retardation syndromes but these changes are without great diagnostic significance. Nevertheless, the presence of pseudoepiphyses may provide a useful hint of wider skeletal involvement when only hand radiographs are available.

2.6.2.3   Dense, Sclerotic Epiphyses

Isolated, single ivory epiphyses occur as a normal variant. They are common in many syndromic associations and occur in patients with chromosomal abnormalities and congenital heart diseases. Ivory epiphyses of the phalanges are a diagnostic feature of Thiemann disease.

2.6.3   Carpus and Tarsus

2.6.3.1   Fusions

Fusions in the carpus and tarsus may be sporadic and idiopathic anatomical variations, or components of skeletal dysplasias, mental retardation/multiple anomalies syndromes and "private" joint contracture syndromes. They usually involve two bones. In some disorders the particular combination of fused bones has diagnostic significance, while in others fusion is non-specific and sometimes progressive.

2.6.3.1.1   *Anatomical Variants (most common fusions; Triquetrum-Lunate; Capitate-Hamate; Trapezium-Scaphoid)*

2.6.3.1.2   *Chondroectodermal Dysplasia (Ellis–van Creveld Syndrome) [Capitate and Hamate Fusion]*

2.6.3.1.3   *Diastrophic Dysplasia*

2.6.3.1.4   *Oto-palato-digital Syndrome (Capitate and Hamate Fusion, Malsegmentation of the Carpal and Tarsal Bones)*

2.6.3.1.5   *Frontometaphyseal Dysplasia (older patients)*

2.6.3.1.6   *Multiple Synostoses Syndrome*

2.6.3.1.7   *Mesomelic Dysplasia (Nievergelt Type)*

2.6.3.1.8   *Acrocephalosyndactyly Syndromes (e.g. Apert Syndrome)*

2.6.3.1.9   *Hand-foot-uterus Syndrome*

2.6.3.1.10   *Arthrogryposis (i.e. Familial Stiff Joint Syndromes with Synostosis)*

2.6.3.1.11   *Spondylo-carpo-tarsal Fusion Syndrome*

2.6.3.1.12   *Holt–Oram Syndrome*

2.6.3.1.13   *Chromosomal Abnormalities*

2.6.3.1.14   *Foetal Alcohol Syndrome*

2.6.3.1.15   *Chronic Rheumatoid Disease*

2.6.3.2   Supernumerary Ossification Centres

The presence of accessory ossification centres in the carpus and/or tarsus is a valuable sign in the recognition of some bone dysplasias. The significance of this finding increases with the age of the patient as the normal and accessory ossicles appear.

2.6.3.2.1   *Anatomical Variants*

2.6.3.2.2   *Larsen Syndrome*

2.6.3.2.3   *Oto-palato-digital Syndrome*

2.6.3.2.4   *Diastrophic Dysplasia*

2.6.3.2.5   *Chondroectodermal Dysplasia (Ellis–van Creveld Syndrome)*

2.6.4   Thumb Abnormalities

2.6.4.1   Thumb Hypoplasia, Aplasia, or Agenesis

Thumb hypoplasia, aplasia, or agenesis has diagnostic value in certain circumstances and the appearance of the thumb should always be carefully evaluated. However, these changes often occur in random association with other clinical abnormalities, in syndromic associations and with bony abnormalities in skeletal dysplasias; their diagnostic value is thereby diminished. In addition, shortening of the distal phalanx of the thumb is present in up to 3% of some population groups, while shortening of the proximal phalanx is a fairly common non-specific variant. Thumb abnormalities are often associated with similar changes in the great toes.
    The thumb is abnormal in the following syndromes:

2.6.4.1.1   Diastrophic Dysplasia (short rigid hitch-hiker thumb)
2.6.4.1.2   Rubinstein–Taybi Syndrome (broad terminal phalanx)
2.6.4.1.3   Fibrodysplasia Ossificans Progressiva (variable hypoplasia)
2.6.4.1.4   Hand-Foot-Uterus Syndrome
2.6.4.1.5   Radial Ray Abnormalities
2.6.4.1.6   Mesomelic Dysplasia (Werner type)
2.6.4.1.7   Cerebro-oculo-facio-skeletal syndrome (Pena–Shokeir Syndrome)
2.6.4.1.8   Popliteal Pterygium Syndrome
2.6.4.1.9   Chromosomal Disorders

2.6.4.2   Finger-like or Triphalangeal Thumb

A finger-like or triphalangeal thumb is a valuable sign in some bone dysostoses and malformation syndromes, but it is of little value in the recognition of bone dysplasias. It can occur in association with other defects and as an isolated, sporadic or familial anomaly. Triphalangy of the big toe is extremely rare.

2.6.4.2.1   Isolated Triphalangy
2.6.4.2.2   Associated with hand and foot abnormalities (e.g. Lobster Claw Foot and Hand)

2.6.4.2.3   Associated with radial hypoplasia (e.g. Radial Hypoplasia/Thrombocytopenia, Fanconi Pancytopenia, Holt–Oram Syndrome)

2.6.4.2.4   Associated with bone marrow dysfunction (e.g. Fanconi Pancytopenia, Blackfan–Diamond Syndrome, Radial Hypoplasia/Thrombocytopenia)

2.6.4.2.5   Associated with congenital heart disease (e.g. Holt–Oram Syndrome)

2.6.4.2.6   Associated with anorectal malformations (e.g. Townes syndrome)

2.6.4.2.7   Associated with onychodystrophy and deafness (e.g. onychodystrophy, distal osteodystrophy and deafness)

2.6.4.2.8   Associated with miscellaneous abnormalities (e.g. Trichorhinophalangeal Syndrome II, acrofacial dysostosis, trisomy 13)

2.6.4.2.9   Associated with maternal teratogen exposure (e.g. Dilantin, Thalidomide)

2.6.4.2.10 Christian Brachydactyly

2.6.4.2.11 Juberg–Hayward Syndrome

2.6.4.2.12 Yunis–Varon Syndrome

2.6.5   Acro-osteolysis (Idiopathic Osteolysis)

The term "acro-osteolysis" denotes progressive disappearance of the peripheral bones. This process may be secondary to neurological disease or osteitis or, less commonly, primary or idiopathic. The idiopathic acro-osteolyses are subclassified as "phalangeal" when the lytic process starts at the periphery and as "carpo-tarsal" when the changes are in the wrists and ankles. Some of the idiopathic, rare acro-osteolysis syndromes have a characteristic radiographic appearance that is much more severe than that of true peripheral acro-osteolysis. Acro-osteolysis should be distinguished from the multicentric osteolyses (see 1.1.4).

In general the radiographic appearances are those of "disappearing bones" and it may be difficult to distinguish the different forms on a single radiograph. Moreover, in the early stages they may mimic the irregular hypoplasia that occurs in genetic skeletal disorders such as cleidocranial dysplasia. Congenital short distal phalanges are seen in brachydactyly B, fetal dilantin syndrome. Keutel syndrome can mimic acroosteolysis.

2.6.5.1   Idiopathic Acro-osteolyses, Predominantly Phalangeal

2.6.5.1.1   Hereditary Acro-osteolysis, Several Forms

2.6.5.1.2   Hadju–Cheney Type

2.6.5.2   Idiopathic Acro-osteolyses, Predominantly Carpo-tarsal

    2.6.5.2.1   Carpo-tarsal Osteolysis with Nephropathy
    2.6.5.2.2   Francois Syndrome (Dermato-corneal Dystrophy)

2.6.5.3   Acro-osteolysis with Neurological Deficit

    2.6.5.3.1   Genetic Conditions
    Acrodystrophic Neuropathy (autosomal dominant)
    Acrodystrophic Neuropathy (autosomal recessive)
    Acrodystrophic Neuropathy (associated with neural
    deafness)
    Congenital indifference to pain
    Charcot–Marie–Tooth Syndrome
    Riley–Day Syndrome (familial dysautonomia)

    2.6.5.3.2   Congenital Non-genetic Conditions
    Syringomyelia
    Myelomeningocele

    2.6.5.3.3   Acquired conditions
    Tabes dorsalis
    Haematomyelia
    Primary amyloid neuropathy
    Diabetic neuropathy
    Pernicious anaemia neuropathy
    Spinal cord trauma
    Peripheral nerve injury
    Yaws
    Leprosy
    Malnutrition (alcoholism or nutritional neuropathy)

2.6.5.4   Acro-osteolysis without Neurological Deficit

    2.6.5.4.1   Genetic Conditions

In the majority of conditions in this category additional changes in other
regions of the skeleton permit definitive diagnosis.

    Dysosteosclerosis
    Cleidocranial Dysplasia
    Complex Carbohydrate Metabolic Disorders (MPS
    and MLS)
    Pachydermoperiostosis (Familial Idiopathic
    Osteoarthropathy)
    Pycnodysostosis
    Singleton–Merten Syndrome
    Progeria
    Werner Syndrome

Rothmund–Thomson Syndrome
Erythropoietic Protoporphyria
Epidermolysis Bullosa Dystrophica
Satoyoshi Syndrome
Hyperparathyroidism

2.6.5.4.2 *Acquired Conditions*
Osteitis
Gout
Juvenile rheumatoid arthritis
Arthritis mutilans (severe rheumatoid arthritis)
Psoriatic arthritis
Ankylosing spondylitis
Scleroderma
Sarcoid
Endangiitis obliterans
Raynaud phenomenon
Sezary syndrome
Vinyl chloride acro-osteolysis
Trauma (electric, frostbite, guitar players, burns)
Dilantin Therapy, long-term

Section 3

Skeletal Dysplasia Syndromes

Summary of Clinical, Radiological, and Genetic Data

Key to Genetic Abbreviations

AD	*Autosomal Dominant*
AR	*Autosomal Recessive*
XL	*X-linked*

In addition to the classical skeletal dysplasias, there are other multi-system disorders in which osseous abnormalities form a significant syndromic component. Conditions of this type that enter into the radiological differential diagnosis of the skeletal dysplasias are included in this section.

The numerical system which is conventionally used to denote specific genetic disorders appears in McKusick's catalogue "Mendelian Inheritance in Man" (MIM). These numbers are quoted and cross-referenced in this section.

Aarskog Syndrome (Faciogenital Dysplasia) [305400]

Clinical features: Stunted stature, round face with hypertelorism, abnormal ears and teeth, stubby digits, shawl scrotum.

Radiographic features: Abnormal vertebrae, especially in the cervical spine, scoliosis, cubitus valgus, metatarsus adductus, mild brachydactyly.

Genetics: XL with partial expression in carrier females.

Other considerations: Clinical features are similar to the Noonan syndrome.

References: Berry C, Cree J, Mann T (1980). Aarskog's syndrome. Arch Dis Child 55:706–710
Porteous MEM and Goudie DR (1991). Aarskog syndrome. J Med Genet 28:44–47

Achondrogenesis Type I (Parenti-Fraccaro) [200600]

Clinical features: Lethal neonatal dwarfism. Gross micromelia, large head, foetal hydrops.

Radiographic features: Tubular bones are very short and dysplastic. Cranium, pelvis and vertebral bodies very poorly ossified. Ribs thin with flared anterior ends.

Genetics: AR (heterogeneous).

Other considerations: Further heterogeneity may exist. The eponym "Houston–Harris" is used for this disorder, which has been sub-grouped into types 1A and 1B [600972], on a basis of their basic defects. The Brazilian or Grebe type of achondrogenesis (now termed Grebe dysplasia [200700]) is a different entity in which survival is usual.

References: Borochowitz Z, Lachman R, Adomian GE, Spear G, Jones K, Rimoin DL (1988). Delineation of further heterogeneity and identification of two distinct sub-groups. J Pediatr 112:23–31
Kozlowski K, Masel J, Morris L, Ryan J, Collins F, Van Vliet P, Woolnough H (1977). Neonatal death dwarfism (report of 17 cases). Australas Radiol 21:164–169

Superti-Furga A, Hastbacka J, Wilcox WR, Cohn DH, van der Harten HJ, Rossi A, Blau N, Rimoin DL, Steinmann B, Lander ES, Gitzelman R (1996). Achondrogenesis type 1B is caused by mutations in the diastrophic dysplasia sulphate transporter gene. Nature Genet 12:100–102

Achondrogenesis Type II (Langer–Saldino Dysplasia) [200610]

Clinical features: Indistinguishable from achondrogenesis type I (*vide supra*).

Radiographic features: Tubular bones are short, with metaphyseal spurs. Ribs short and stubby. Iliac bones normal. Vertebral bodies under-ossified. Cranial vault normal.

Genetics: AD (new dominant mutation).

Other considerations: Specific radiographic stigmata permit differentiation between Types I and II. Type II Achondrogenesis is the result of a mutation in the type II collagen gene, and it is regarded as part of a spectrum which also embraces hypochondrogenesis [120140.0007].

References: Chen H, Liu CT, Yang SS (1981). Achondrogenesis: a review with special consideration of achondrogenesis type II (Langer–Saldino). Am J Med Genet 10:379–394

Rittler M, Orioli IM (1995). Achondrogenesis type II with polydactyly. Am J Med Genet 59:157–160

Whitley CB, Gorlin RJ (1983). Achondrogenesis: New nosology with evidence of genetic heterogeneity. Radiology 148:693–698

Achondroplasia [100800]

Clinical features: Rhizomelic dwarfism, characteristic facies with large head and depressed nasal bridge, trident hand. Spinal complications in adulthood.

Radiographic features: Shortening of the base of the skull with small foramen magnum, shortening of the tubular bones with metaphyseal flaring, small sacro-iliac notches, narrowing of the lumbar spinal canal, progressive caudal interpedicular narrowing.

Genetics: AD.

Other considerations: Achondroplasia is by far the most common form of short-limbed dwarfism.

References: Lachman RS (1997). Neurologic abnormalities in the skeletal dysplasias: a clinical and radiological perspective. Am J Med Genet 69:33–43

Langer LO Jr, Baumann PA, Gorlin RJ (1967) Achondroplasia. Am J Roentgenol 100:12–26

Pauli RM, Horton VK, Glinksi LP, Reiser CA (1995). Prospective assessment of risks for cervicomedullary-junction compression in infants with achondroplasia. Am J Hum Genet 56:732–744

Acrocephalopolysyndactyly Type II (see Carpenter Syndrome)

Acrocephalosyndactyly (see Apert Syndrome)

Acrodysostosis [101800]

Clinical features: Short stature, mental retardation, peculiar facies, stubby extremities.

Radiographic features: Shortening of the tubular bones of the hands and feet, premature fusion of cone-shaped epiphyses. Other non-diagnostic skeletal changes.

Genetics: Probably heterogeneous, AD in some families.

Other considerations: Probably underdiagnosed.

References: Butler MG, Rames LJ, Wadlington WB (1988). Acrodysostosis: report of a 13-year old boy with review of literature and metacarpophalangeal pattern profile analysis. Am J Med Genet 30:971–980.

Opitz JM, Mollica F, Sorge G, Milana G, Cimino G, Caltabiano M (1993). Acrofacial dysostoses: review and report of a previously undescribed condition: The autosomal or X-linked dominant Catania form of acrofacial dysostosis. Am J Med Genet 47:660–678

Viljoen D, Beighton P (1991). Epiphyseal stippling in acrodysostosis. Am J Med Genet 38:43–45

Acrodysplasia with Exostoses (see Trichorhinophalangeal Dysplasia)

Acrodysplasia with Retinitis Pigmentosa and Nephropathy (see Saldino–Mainzer Syndrome)

Acromesomelic Dysplasia (see Mesomelic Dysplasia)

Acromicric Dysplasia [102370]

Clinical features:	Stunted stature, flexed digits, unusual facies.
Radiographic features:	Dysplastic femoral capital epiphyses, cone-shaped phalangeal epiphyses, proximal pointing of meta-carpals.
Genetics:	AD?
Other considerations:	Very rare.
References:	Maroteaux P, Stanescu R, Stanescu V, Rappaport R (1986). Acromicric dysplasia. Am J Med Genet 24:447–459

Acro-osteolysis Syndromes (see Osteolysis Syndromes)

Adams–Oliver Syndrome

Clinical features:	Reduction defects of digits, sometimes extending to involve the distal portions of the limbs. Ulcerated scalp defects, which heal with scarring, may be present at birth.
Radiographic features:	Hypoplasia of the tubular bones of the extremities. Defects of the calvarium underlying the scalp lesions.
Genetics:	AD.
Other considerations:	There is nosological confusion with the ectrodactyly, ectodermal dysplasia, facial clefts syndrome (EEC [129900]) and the Split Hand-Split Foot malformation [183600].

References: Bonafede P, Beighton P (1979). Autosomal
                          dominant inheritance of scalp defects with
                          ectrodactyly. Am J Med Genet 3:35–41
                          Bamforth JS, Kaurah P, Byrne J, Ferreira P (1994).
                          Adams Oliver syndrome: a family with extreme
                          variability in clinical expression. Am J Med
                          Genet 49:393–396
                          Klinger G, Merlob P (1998). Adams–Oliver
                          syndrome: autosomal recessive inheritance
                          and new phenotypic–anthropometric findings.
                          Am J Med Genet 79:197–199
                          Kuster W, Lenz W, Kaariainen H, Majewski F
                          (1988). Congenital scalp defects with distal
                          limb anomalies (Adams–Oliver syndrome):
                          report of ten cases and review of the literature.
                          Am J Med Genet 31:99–115

Adenosine Deaminase Deficiency [102700]

Clinical features: Failure to thrive with death from recurrent infec-
                          tions during infancy, immunodeficiency, flared
                          bone ends.

Radiographic features: Widening and cupping of the metaphyses and
                          costochondral junctions.

Genetics: AR.

Other considerations: This rare, but lethal, condition was among the
                          first to be treated at the molecular level by gene
                          therapy.

References: Bordignon C, Notarangelo LD, Nobili N, Ferrari
                          G, Casorati G, Panina P, Mazzolari E, Maggioni
                          D, Rossi C, Servida P, Ugazio AG, Mavilio F
                          (1995). Gene therapy in peripheral blood lym-
                          phocytes and bone marrow for ADA: immuno-
                          deficient patients. Science 270:470–475
                          Cedarbaum SD, Kaitila J, Rimoin DL, Stiehm ER
                          (1976). The chondro-osseous dysplasia of ADA
                          deficiency with severe combined immuno-
                          deficiency. J Pediat 89:737–747

Aicardi Syndrome [304050]

Clinical features: Mental retardation, infantile spasms, chorio-

	retinal lacunae, agenesis of the corpus callosum, specific EEG changes.
Radiographic features:	Localised mild malsegmentation of the spine.
Genetics:	X-linked dominant with male lethality (?).
Other considerations:	The majority of reports concern affected females.
References:	Besenski N, Bosnjak V, Ligutia I, Marusic-Della Marina B (1988). Cortical heterotopia in Aicardi's syndrome – CT findings. Pediatr Radiol 18:391–393
	Phillips HE, Carter AP, Kennedy JL, Rosman NP, O'Connor JF (1978). Aicardi's syndrome: radiologic manifestations. Radiology 127:453–455
	Trifiletti RR, Incorpora G, Polizzi A, Cocuzza MD, Bolan EA, Parano E (1995). Aicardi syndrome with multiple tumors: a case report with literature review. Brain Dev 17:283–285

Alagille Syndrome (see Arteriohepatic Dysplasia)

Albright Hereditary Osteodystrophy
(see Pseudohypoparathyroidism)

Alkaptonuria [203500]

Clinical features:	Widespread degenerative arthropathy, especially of the spine. Black pigmentation in cartilage, including the pinnae of the ears and the sclerae. Dark urine.
Radiographic features:	Degenerative changes in the spine and large joints. Intra-articular loose bodies. Synchondrosis of the pubis.
Genetics:	AR.
Other considerations:	The term "ochronosis" is descriptive of dark pigmentation of connective tissue, which may also be caused by poisoning with phenol. Alkaptonuria is well recognised but has a patchy geographical distribution.
References:	Fernandez-Canon JM, Granadino B, Beltran-Valero de Bernabe D, Renedo M, Fernandez-Ruiz E, Penalva MA, Rodriguez de Cordoba S

(1996). The molecular basis of alkaptonuria. Nature Genet 14:19–24

Justesen P, Anderson PE (1984). Radiologic manifestations in alcaptonuria. Skeletal Radiol 11:204–208

O'Brien WM, La Du BN, Bunim JJ (1963). Biochemical, pathologic and clinical aspects of alcaptonuria, ochronosis and ochronotic arthropathy: review of the world literature. Am J Med 34:813–818

Angio-osteohypertrophy (see Klippel–Trenaunay–Weber Syndrome)

Apert Syndrome (Acrocephalosyndactyly) [101200]

Clinical features:

Turricephaly, syndactyly (mitten hands and feet), mental retardation.

Radiographic features:

Craniostenosis, phalangeal dysplasia and fusion.

Genetics:

AD, but the majority of affected persons have normal parents and represent new mutations.

Other considerations:

Several other acrocephalosyndactyly syndromes bearing eponyms such as "Vogt" and "Pfeiffer" differ by virtue of the severity of their cranial and digital involvement; there is controversy concerning their precise identity.

References:

Cohen MM, Kreiborg S (1993). Skeletal abnormalities in the Apert syndrome. Am J Med Genet 47:624–632

Cohen MM Jr, Kreiborg S (1995). Hands and feet in the Apert syndrome. Am J Med Genet 57:82–96

Kreiborg S, Barr M Jr., Cohen MM Jr. (1992). Cervical spine in the Apert syndrome. Am J Med Genet 43:704–708

Arteriohepatic Dysplasia (Alagille Syndrome) [118450]

Clinical features:

Hepatic disease, cholestasis, pulmonary artery stenosis, retarded physical, mental and sexual development, characteristic facies.

Radiographic features: Mild localised vertebral malsegmentation. "Butterfly" vertebral configuration.

Genetics: AD.

Other considerations: Rare.

References: Alagille D, Estrada A, Hadchouel M, Gautier M, Odievre M, Dommergues JP (1987). Syndromic paucity of interlobular bile ducts (Alagille syndrome or arteriohepatic dysplasia): Review of 80 cases. J Pediatr 110:195–200

Brunelle F, Estrada A, Dommergues JP, Bernard O, Chaumont P (1986). Skeletal anomalies in Alagille's syndrome. Radiographic study in 80 cases. Ann Radiol (Paris) 29:687–690

Krantz ID, Piccoli DA, Spinner NB (1997). Alagille syndrome. J Med Genet 34:152–157

Arthrogryposis

Clinical features: Multiple congenital contractures.

Radiographic features: Gracile bones.

Genetics: Common form is non-genetic, others very heterogeneous.

Other considerations: The term "arthrogryposis" is often used loosely for any disorder in which articular rigidity is present at birth. Apart from the relatively common non-genetic condition "amyoplasia" or classical arthrogryposis multiplex congenita, there are many rare inherited stiff joint syndromes. These differ in their pathogenesis and mode of transmission.

References: Hall JG, Reed SD, Greene G (1982). The distal arthrogryposes: delineation of new entities: review with nosologic discussion. Am J Med Genet 11:185–246

Krakowiak PA, O'Quinn JR, Bohnsack JF, Watkins WS, Carey JC, Jorde LB, Bamshad M (1997). A variant of Freeman–Sheldon syndrome maps to 11p15.5-pter. Am J Hum Genet 60:426–432

Poznanski AK, La Rowe PC (1970). Radiographic manifestations of the arthrogryposis syndrome. Radiology 95:353–358

Arthro-ophthalmopathy (Stickler Syndrome) [108300]

Clinical features:	Marfanoid habitus, myopia, cleft palate, micrognathia, generalised arthropathy.
Radiographic features:	Mild platyspondyly with generalised dysplasia of the epiphyses, premature degenerative osteo-arthropathy.
Genetics:	AD with variable expression.
Other considerations:	The type II collagen gene is faulty in some affected families but not in others [184840].
References:	Ballo R, Beighton PH, Ramesar RS (1998). Stickler-like syndrome due to a dominant negative mutation in the COL2A1 gene. Am J Med Genet 80:6–11
	Opitz JM, Franc T. Herrmann J (1972). The Stickler syndrome. N Engl J Med 286:546–547.
	Vintiner GM, Temple IK, Middleton-Price HR, Baraitser M, Malcolm S (1991). Genetic and clinical heterogeneity of Stickler syndrome. Am J Med Genet 41:44–48
	Winter RM, Baraitser M, Laurence KM, Donnai D, Hall CM (1983). The Weissenbacher–Zweymül-ler, Stickler, and Marshall syndromes: further evidence for their identity. Am J Med Genet 16:189–199

Aspartylglucosaminuria (see Complex Carbohydrate Metabolic Disorders)

Asphyxiating Thoracic Dysplasia (Jeune Syndrome) [208500]

Clinical features:	Narrow thorax, shortened extremities, post-axial polydactyly. Often fatal in the newborn. Renal complications may develop in late childhood in survivors.

Radiographic features: Short ribs, triradiate acetabulae, premature ossification of capital femoral epiphyses, minor metaphyseal changes, cone-shaped epiphyses.

Genetics: AR, heterogeneous (?).

Other considerations: Respiratory and renal complications are inconsistent and may be indicative of heterogeneity.

References: Cortina H, Beltran J, Olague R, Ceres L, Alonso A, Lanuza A (1979). The wide spectrum of the asphyxiating thoracic dysplasia. Pediatr Radiol 8:93–99

Kozlowski K, Masel J (1976). Asphyxiating thoracic dystrophy without respiratory distress. J Pediatr Radiol 5:30–33

Nagai T, Nishimura G, Kato R, Hasegawa T, Ohashi H, Fukushima Y (1995). Del(12)(p11.21p12.2) associated with an asphyxiating thoracic dystrophy or chondroectodermal dysplasia-like syndrome. Am J Med Genet 55:16–18

Atelosteogenesis Type I (Spondylo-humero-femoral Hypoplasia) [108720]

Clinical features: Lethal micromelic neonatal dwarfism with incurved legs, clubfeet, dislocated elbows and inconsistent cleft palate.

Radiographic features: Incomplete ossification and coronal clefts of the lumbar vertebrae with hypoplasia of the upper thoracic vertebral bodies. The humerus and femur are club-shaped with distal hypoplasia. Lack of ossification of single phalanges and metacarpals is often evident.

Genetics: AD, new mutation?

Other considerations: The condition is subdivided into type I and type II; the latter was formerly known as de la Chapelle dysplasia (*vide infra*). A type III has also been proposed [108721].

References: Kozlowski K, Tsuruta T, Kameda Y, Kan A, Leslie G (1981). New forms of neonatal death dwarfism. Report of 3 cases. Pediatr Radiol 10:155–160

Maroteaux P, Spranger J, Stanescu V, Le Marec B, Pfeiffer RA, Beighton P, Mattei JF (1982). Atelosteogenesis. Am J Med Genet 13:15–25

Schultz C, Langer LO, Laxova R, Pauli RN (1999). Atelosteogenesis Type III: long term survival, prenatal diagnosis, and evidence for dominant transmission. Am J Med Genet 83:28–42

Stern HJ, Graham JM Jr, Lachman RS, Horton W, Bernini PM, Spiegel PK, Bodurtha J, Ives EJ, Bocian M, Rimoin DL (1990). Atelosteogenesis type III: a distinct skeletal dysplasia with features overlapping atelosteogenesis and oto-palato-digital syndrome type II. Am J Med Genet 36:183–195

Atelosteogenesis Type II (de la Chapelle Dysplasia) [256050]

Clinical Features: Lethal neonatal dwarfism with gross limb shortening.

Radiographic features: Unique and unmistakable triangular configuration of fibula and ulna.

Genetics: AR.

Other considerations: Very rare. Initially termed "de la Chapelle dysplasia". Now regarded as a form of atelosteogenesis and also termed neonatal osseous dysplasia. The molecular defect is similar to that of diastrophic dysplasia.

References:

Rossi A, van der Harten HJ, Beemer FA, Kleijer WJ, Gitzelmann R, Steinmann B, Superti-Furga A (1996). Phenotypic and genotypic overlap between atelosteogenesis type 2 and diastrophic dysplasia. Hum Genet 98:657–661

Sillence D, Kozlowski K, Rogers J, Sprague P, Cullity G, Osborn R (1987). Atelosteogenesis: evidence for heterogeneity. Pediat Radiol 17:112–118

Whitley CB, Burke BA, Granroth G, Gorlin RJ (1986). De la Chapelle dysplasia. Am J Med Genet 25:229–239

Baller–Gerold Syndrome (see Craniosynostosis with Radial Defects)

Basal Cell Naevus Carcinoma Syndrome [109400]

Clinical features:	Basal cell naevi that are prone to become carcinomatous. Mild mental deficiency, characteristic facies.
Radiographic features:	Intracranial calcifications, mandibular cysts, malsegmentation of the ribs, short metacarpals.
Genetics:	AD.
Other considerations:	The bony changes are overshadowed by the dermal lesions.
References:	Gorlin RJ (1987). Nevoid basal-cell carcinoma syndrome. Medicine 66:98–113
	Kimonis VE, Goldstein AM, Pastakia B, Yang ML, Kase R, DiGiovanna JJ, Bale AE, Bale SJ (1997). Clinical manifestations in 105 persons with nevoid basal cell carcinoma syndrome. Am J Med Genet 69:299–308
	Kozlowski K, Baker P, Glasson M (1974). Multiple nevoid basal cell carcinoma syndrome. Pediatr Radiol 2:185–190.
	Lo Muzio L, Nocini PF, Savoia A, Consolo U, Procaccini M, Zelante L, Pannone G, Bucci P, Dolci M, Bambini F, Solda P, Favia G (1999). Nevoid basal cell carcinoma syndrome. Clinical findings in 37 Italian affected individuals. Clin Genet 55:34–40

Beckwith–Wiedemann Syndrome [130650]

Clinical features:	Excessive growth, peculiar facies, large tongue and exomphalos.
Radiographic features:	Accelerated bone age.
Genetics:	AD with variable expression. Heterogeneous?
Other considerations:	The stigmata vary in degree and definitive diagnosis may be difficult. The genetic mechanism of "imprinting" may be operative.

References: Lam WWK, Hatada I, Ohishi S, Mukai T, Joyce JA, Cole TRP, Donnai D, Reik W, Schofield PN, Maher ER (1999). Analysis of germline CDKN1C (p57KIP2) mutations in familial and sporadic Beckwith-Wiedemann syndrome (BWS) provides a novel genotype–phenotype correlation. J Med Genet 36:518–523
Lee FA (1972). Radiology of the Beckwith–Wiedemann syndrome. Radiol Clin North Am 10:261–276
Pettenati MJ, Haines JL, Higgins RR, Wappner RS, Palmer CG (1986). Wiedemann–Beckwith syndrome: presentation of clinical and cytogenetic data on 22 new cases and review of the literature. Hum Genet 74:143–154
Weng EY, Moeschler JB, Graham JM Jr (1995). Longitudinal observations on 15 children with Wiedemann–Beckwith syndrome. Am J Med Genet 56:366–373

Beemer-Langer Syndrome (see Short Rib Syndrome Type IV)

Beta-Glucuronidase Deficiency; MPS VII (see Dysostosis Multiplex group; Complex Carbohydrate Metabolic Disorders)

Binder Syndrome (Maxillonasal Dysplasia) [155050]

Clinical features: Stunted stature, flat nasal bridge, very short nasal columella, stubby terminal phalanges.

Radiographic features: Epiphyseal stippling in infancy in some instances. Hypoplasia of terminal phalanges. Occasional vertebral fusion or clefting.

Genetics: Unknown. Heterogeneous?

Other considerations: There is nosological confusion with acrodysostosis and with mild forms of chondrodysplasia punctata. An AR form of frontonasal dysostosis with polysyndactyly and tibial hypoplasia has been documented.

References: Quarrell OWJ, Koch M, Hughes HE (1990) Maxillonasal dysplasia (Binder's syndrome). J Med Genet 27:384–387

Olow-Nordenran M, Valentin J (1984) Maxillo-nasal dysplasia (Binder syndrome) and associated malformations of the cervical spine. Acta Radiol 25:353–360

Slaney SF, Goodman FR, Eilers-Walsman BLC, Hall BD, Williams DK, Young ID, Hayward RD, Jones BM, Christianson AL. Winter RM (1999). Acromelic frontonasal dysostosis. Am J Med Genet 83:109–116

Bird-headed Dwarfism (see Seckel Syndrome)

Blount Disease [259200]

Clinical features: Bow legs and tibial torsion developing when walking commences (infantile type) or at the end of the first decade (late type).

Radiographic features: Flattening of the medial side of the upper tibial and lower femoral epiphyses and metaphyses. Late Blount disease, which may be asymmetrical, is the consequence of the collapse of the medial side of the upper tibial plateau.

Genetics: Non-genetic.

Other considerations: The early form of Blount disease, which has a predilection for persons of indigenous African stock, may represent exaggerated and progressive physiological bowing of infancy. The late form results from infection, trauma or unresolved early Blount disease.

References: Bathfield CA, Beighton P (1978). Blount disease: a review of aetiological factors in 110 patients. Clin Orthop 135:29–33

Mitchell EI, Chung SMK, Das MM, Gregg JR (1980). A new radiographic grading system for Blount disease, evaluating the epiphyseal metaphyseal angle. Orthop Rev 9:27–33

Boomerang Dysplasia [1123103]

Clinical features: Lethal neonatal short-limbed dwarfism, with rigid limbs, a broad nasal root and hypoplasia of the nares and septum.

Radiographic features: Absence of radii and fibulae; other long bones
                           have a curved "boomerang" configuration. Iliac
                           bones are small and ossification in the lower spine
                           and digits is retarded.

Genetics: XL?

Other considerations: All reported cases have been male. An aetiological
                           relationship with atelosteogenesis has been pro-
                           posed.

References: Kozlowski K, Sillence D, Cortis-Jones R, Osborn R
                           (1985). Case report: Boomerang dysplasia Br J
                           Radiol 369–371
                           Odent S, Loget P, Le Marec B, Delezoïde AL,
                           Maroteaux P (1999). Unusual fan shaped
                           ossification in a female fetus with radiological
                           features of boomerang dysplasia. J Med Genet
                           36:330–332
                           Oostra RJ, Dijkstra PF, Baljet B, Verbeeten BWJM,
                           Hennekam RCM (1999). A 100-year old ana-
                           tomical specimen presenting with boomerang-
                           like skeletal dysplasia: diagnostic strategies and
                           outcome. Am J Med Genet 85:134–139
                           Winship I, Cremin B, Beighton P (1990). Boom-
                           erang dysplasia. Am J Med Genet 36:440–443.

Brachydactyly Syndromes [112500; 113000; 133100]

Clinical features: Stubby hands and feet. A wide variety of addition-
                           al stigmata may be present.

Radiographic features: Short tubular bones of the hands and feet with
                           cone-shaped epiphyses.

Genetics: AD, very heterogeneous.

Other considerations: Numerous brachydactyly syndromes have been
                           delineated. The pattern of digital involvement or
                           the presence of other anomalies permits diagnos-
                           tic precision. The classical forms of isolated
                           brachydactyly are designated types "A–E".
                           Angel-shaped phalango-epiphyseal dysplasia
                           (ASPED) [105835] and Brachydactyly-hyperten-
                           sion dysplasia [112410] are other disorders in this
                           category.

References: Fitch N (1979). Classification and identification of
                                 inherited brachydactylies. J Med Genet 16:36–
                                 44
                                 Sharma AK, Haldar A, Phadke SR, Agarwal SS
                                 (1994). Preaxial brachydactyly with abduction
                                 of thumbs and hallux varus: a distinct entity.
                                 Am J Med Genet 49:274–277.
                                 Temtamy SA, McKusick VA (1978). The genetics
                                 of hand malformations. New York: Alan R Liss

Brachyolmia (Short Spine Dysplasia) [113500; 271530]

Clinical features: Short trunked dwarfism.

Radiographic features: Platyspondyly, short dysplastic femoral necks; the
                                 skeleton is otherwise normal.

Genetics: AD/AR.

Other considerations: In view of the involvement of the upper femoral
                                 metaphyseal region, some experts consider that
                                 brachyolmia should be regarded as a spondylo-
                                 metaphyseal dysplasia.

References: Gardner J, Beighton P (1994). Brachyolmia: auto-
                                 somal dominant form. Am J Med Genet 49:308–
                                 312.
                                 Horton WA, Langer LO, Collins DL, Dwyer C
                                 (1983). Brachyolmia, recessive type (Hobaek): a
                                 clinical, radiographic and histochemical study.
                                 Am J Med Genet 16:201–211
                                 Shohat M, Lachman R, Gruber HE, Rimoin DL
                                 (1989). Brachyolmia: radiographic and genetic
                                 evidence of heterogeneity. Am J Med Genet
                                 33:209–219

Bruck Syndrome (see Osteogenesis Imperfecta with Congenital Contractures)

Buschke–Ollendorff Syndrome (see Osteopoikilosis)

Caffey Disease (Infantile Cortical Hyperostosis) [114000]

Clinical features: Inflammation and swelling of the mandible which
                                 develops in infancy and resolves spontaneously.

The shoulder girdle and tubular bones are sometimes involved.

Radiographic features: Hyperostosis and new bone formation, producing irregular widening of the cortices of the affected bones.

Genetics: AD(?), Non-genetic form (?).

Other considerations: The aetiology is unknown, but familial clustering and sporadic outbreaks have been reported. Antenatal diagnosis has been documented.

References: de Jongh G, Muller LMM (1995). Perinatal death in two sibs with infantile cortical hyperostosis (Caffey disease). Am J Med Genet 59:134–138

Faure C, Beyssac JM, Montagne JP (1977). Predominant or exclusive orbital and facial involvement in infantile cortical hyperostosis (de Toni–Caffey's disease). Report of 4 cases and a review of the literature. Pediatr Radiol 6:103–108

Borochowitz A, Gozal D, Misselevitch I, Aunallah J, Boss JH (1991). Familial Caffey's disease and late recurrence in a child. Clin Genet 40:329–335

Campanacci Syndrome (see Osteofibrous Dysplasia of the Tibia and Fibula)

Campomelic Dysplasia [211970]

Clinical features: Neonatal dwarfism, anterolateral bowing of the legs, talipes equinovarus, tracheobronchomalacia. The phenotypic and chromosomal sex may be incongruous.

Radiographic features: Shortening and bowing of the long bones, especially the fibula. Hypoplastic iliac bones and scapulae. Hip dislocation, thin ribs, hypoplasia of the cervical spine.

Genetics: AR. Heterogeneous.

Other considerations: In the AR Cumming type [211890] a cervical lymphocele and polycystic organ dysplasia are additional features. An AD form [114290] has been proposed.

References: Dibbern KM, Graham JM, Lachman RS, Wilcox WR (1998). Cumming syndrome: report of two additional cases. Pediatr Radiol 28:798–801

Kozlowski K, Butzer HO, Galatus-Jensen F, Tulloch A (1978). Syndromes of congenital bowing of the long bones. Pediatr Radiol 7:40–48

Mansour S, Hall CM, Pembrey ME, Young ID (1995). A clinical and genetic study of campomelic dysplasia. J Med Genet 32:415–420

Pérez del Río MJ, Fernández-Toral J, Madrigal B, González-González M, Ablanedo P, Herrero A (1999). Two new cases of Cumming syndrome confirming autosomal recessive inheritance. Am J Med Genet 82:340–343

Camurati–Engelmann Disease (see Diaphyseal Dysplasia)

Carpenter Syndrome (Acrocephalopolysyndactyly Type II) [201000]

Clinical features: High domed forehead, syndactyly, pre-axial polydactyly and structural cardiac defects.

Radiographic features: Craniostenosis, duplicated proximal phalanx of the thumb, syndactyly.

Genetics: AR.

Other considerations: Several rare disorders including the Goodman and Summitt syndromes have similar stigmata.

References: Cohen DM, Green JG, Miller J, Gorlin RJ, Reed JA (1987). Acrocephalopolysyndactyly type II – Carpenter syndrome: clinical spectrum and an attempt at unification with Goodman and Summitt syndromes. Am J Med Genet 28:311–324

Gershoni-Baruch R (1990). Carpenter syndrome: marked variability of expression to include the Summitt and Goodman syndromes. Am J Med Genet 35:236–240

Cartilage-Hair Hypoplasia (see Metaphyseal Chondroplasia, McKusick Type)

Cephaloskeletal Dysplasia (see Taybi–Linder Syndrome)

Cerebral Gigantism (Sotos Syndrome) [117550]

Clinical features:	Prenatal onset of excessive size, macrocephaly, peculiar facies, mental retardation, premature eruption of teeth.
Radiographic features:	Advanced bone age commensurate with height.
Genetics:	AD(?).
Other considerations:	Metacarpophalangeal pattern profile analysis may be helpful in diagnostic confirmation.
References:	Allanson JE, Cole TRP (1996). Sotos syndrome: evolution of facial phenotype subjective and objective assessment. Am J Med Genet 65:13–20
	Cole TRP, Hughes HE (1994). Sotos syndrome: a study of the diagnostic criteria and natural history. J Med Genet 31:20–32.
	Winship IM (1985). Sotos syndrome – autosomal dominant inheritance substantiated. Clin Genet 28:243–246

Cerebro-costo-mandibular Syndrome [117650]

Clinical features:	Respiratory distress usually leads to discovery of the disorder. Micrognathia, cleft palate and glossoptosis are the only obvious clinical features. Death in infancy is frequent.
Radiographic features:	Severe micrognathia, bilateral posterior rib gaps.
Genetics:	AD(?).
Other considerations:	Rare.
References:	Hennekam RCM, Goldschmeding R (1998). Complete absence of rib ossification, micrognathia and ear anomalies: extreme expression of cerebro-costo-mandibular syndrome? Eur J Hum Genet 6:71–74

Kirk EPE, Arbuckle S, Ramm PL, Adès LC (1999). Severe micrognathia, cleft palate, absent olfactory tract, and abnormal rib development: cerebro-costo-mandibular syndrome or a new syndrome? Am J Med Genet 84:120–124

Plotz FB, van Essen AJ, Bosschaart AN, Bos AP (1996). Cerebro-costo-mandibular syndrome. Am J Med Genet 62:286–292

Cerebro-hepato-renal Syndrome (Zellweger Syndrome) [214100]

Clinical features: Hypotonia, contractures, peculiar facies, corneal opacities, glaucoma, enlarged liver, mental retardation. Fatal in infancy.

Radiographic features: Extensive granular calcifications of the patellae. Other calcifications similar to those of the dominant form of chondrodysplasia punctata.

Genetics: AR.

Other considerations: Perioxysome biogenesis is faulty in this disorder.

References: Moser AB, Rasmussen M, Naidu S et al. (1995). Phenotype of patients with peroxisomal disorders subdivided into sixteen complementation groups. J Pediat 127:13–22

Williams P (1972). Roentgenographic features of the cerebrohepatorenal syndrome of Zellweger. Am J Roentgenol 115:607–611

Wilson GN, Holmes RG, Custer J, Lipkowitz JL, Stover J, Datta N, Hajra A (1986). Zellweger syndrome: diagnostic assays, syndrome delineation, and potential therapy. Am J Med Genet 24:69–82

Cerebro-oculo-facio-skeletal (COFS) Syndrome (Pena–Shokeir Syndrome) [214150]

Clinical features: Failure to thrive, microphthalmia, characteristic facies, articular contractures, foot deformity.

Radiographic features: Multiple bony ankyloses, contractures, vertical talus, intracranial calcification.

Genetics: AR.

Other considerations: Two forms of this disorder, both bearing the same eponym, have been described. Separate syndromic identity is questionable.

References: Linna SL, Finni K, Simila S, Kouvalainen K, Laitinen J (1982). Intracranial calcification in cerebro-oculo-facio-skeletal (COFS) syndrome. Pediatr Radiol 12:28–30

Pena SDJ, Shokeir MHK (1974). Syndrome of camptodactyly, multiple ankyloses, facial anomalies and pulmonary hypoplasia: a lethal condition. J Pediatr 85:373–378

Temtamy SA, Meguid NA, Mahmoud A, Afifi HH, Gerzawy A, Zaki MS (1996). COFS syndrome with familial 1,16 translocation. Clin Genet 50:240–243

Cervico-oculo-acoustic Syndrome (Wildervanck Syndrome) [314600]

Clinical features: Neck rigidity, unilateral retrusion of the eyeball, sixth nerve palsy and perceptive deafness.

Radiographic features: Fusion of cervical vertebrae.

Genetics: Female preponderance, polygenic or sex-linked dominant with male lethality?

Other considerations: Differs from the Klippel–Feil syndrome by virtue of the additional ocular abnormalities and hearing defect.

References: Schild JA, Mafee MF, Miller MF (1984). Wildervanck syndrome – the external appearance and radiologic findings. Int J Pediatr Otorhinolaryngol 7:305–310

Wildervanck LS, Hoefsema PE, Penning L (1966). Radiological examination of the inner ear of deaf-mutes presenting with the cervico-oculo-acusticus syndrome. Acta Otolaryngol (Stock) 61:445–450

Cheirolumbar Dysostosis

Clinical features: Low back pain and sciatica. Stubby digits.

Radiographic features:	Brachycheiry (shortening of the tubular bones of the hands and feet) with stenosis of the lumbar spinal canal.
Genetics:	AD (?).
Other considerations:	More than 30 cases are known and it is possible that the condition is underdiagnosed.
References:	Wachenheim A (1981). Cheirolumbar dysostosis. Eur J Radiol 1(3):189–194

Cherubism (Fibrous Dysplasia of the Jaws) [118400]

Clinical features:	Swelling of the jaws in early childhood with stasis or regression at puberty. Dental abnormalities.
Radiographic features:	Bilateral, radiolucent defects in the mandible, malposition of the teeth.
Genetics:	AD.
Other considerations:	Cherubism is rare. Most affected persons present with dental or faciomaxillary cosmetic problems. An AR form of Cherubism is associated with gingival fibromatosis [135300].
References:	Sherman NH, Rao VM, Brennan RE, Edeiken J (1982). Fibrous dysplasia of the facial bones and mandible. Skeletal Radiol 8(2):141–143 Wackerle B, Reiser M, Herzog M, Kahn T (1987). Radiologic findings in cherubism: Orthopantomography, CT, MRI. Rontgenpraxis 40:104–107 Yamaguchi T, Dorfman HD, Eisig S (1999). Cherubism: clinicopathological features. Skeletal Radiol 28:350–353

Chondrodysplasia Punctata (Conradi–Hünermann Type) [118650]

Clinical features:	Asymmetry of the extremities, flat face, depressed nasal bridge, ichthyosis, variable progressive spinal malalignment.
Radiographic features:	Asymmetrical shortening of the tubular bones, punctate calcifications, malsegmentation of the spine, kyphoscoliosis.

Genetics: AD. The nosology of chondrodysplasia punctata
                            is complicated; XL dominant [302950] and XL
                            recessive [302940] forms are recognised.

Other considerations: The term "stippled epiphyses" has been used for
                            this disorder but this descriptive designation is
                            also applicable to a number of conditions in
                            which punctate epiphyseal changes are present in
                            infancy.

References: Anderson PE, Justesen P (1987). Chondrodyspla-
                            sia punctata. Skeletal Radiol 16:223–226
                            Happle R (1979). X-linked dominant chondro-
                            dysplasia: review of the literature and report of
                            a case. Hum Genet 53:65–73
                            Maroteaux   P   (1989).   Brachytelephalangic
                            chondrodysplasia punctata: a possible X-linked
                            recessive form. Hum Gen 82:167–170
                            Rittler M, Menger H, Spranger J (1990). Chondro-
                            dysplasia punctata, tibia-metacarpal type. Am J
                            Med Genet 37:200–208
                            Sutphen R, Amar MJ, Kousseff BG, Toomey KE
                            (1995). XXY male with X-linked dominant
                            chondrodysplasia   punctata   (Happle   syn-
                            drome). Am J Med Genet 57:489–492

Chondrodysplasia Punctata, Rhizomelic Form [215100]

Clinical features: Dwarfism with marked rhizomelic shortening of
                            the extremities, ichthyotic skin changes, cataracts,
                            multiple joint contractures, usually lethal in the
                            first year of life. Dislocation of C1–2 may occur.

Radiographic features: Calcific stippling of the epiphyses, tubular bone
                            shortening, especially of the humeri, coronal cleft
                            vertebrae.

Genetics: AR.

Other considerations: This perioxysomal disorder is a rare but well
                            recognised form of potentially lethal dwarfism.
                            Differential diagnosis from other disorders with
                            epiphyseal stippling, including warfarin embryo-
                            pathy, is crucial for accurate prognostication and
                            genetic counselling.

References: Agamanolis DP, Novak RW (1995). Rhizomelic
                              chondrodysplasia punctata: Report of a case
                              with review of the literature and correlation
                              with other peroxisomal disorders. Pediat
                              Pathol Lab Med 15:503–513
                              Gilbert EF, Opitz JM, Spranger JW, Langer LO,
                              Wolfson JJ, Visekul C (1976). Chondrodyspla-
                              sia punctata, rhizomelic form. Eur J Pediatr
                              123(2):89–96
                              Heselson NG, Cremin BJ, Beighton P (1978).
                              Lethal chondrodysplasia punctata. Clin Radiol
                              29:679–684

Chondroectodermal Dysplasia (Ellis–van Creveld Syndrome) [225500]

Clinical features: Short limb dwarfism, polydactyly, hypoplastic
                             nails, dental abnormalities, cardiac defects.

Radiographic features: Narrow thorax, triradiate acetabulum, premature
                             ossification of femoral capital epiphyses, fusion of
                             the carpal bones, cone-shaped epiphyses, charac-
                             teristic shape of the tibia.

Genetics: AR.

Other considerations: The majority of affected persons have been
                             members of the Amish community, a religious
                             isolate in the United States.

References: Kozlowski K, Szmigiel C, Barylak A, Stropyrowa
                             M (1972). Difficulties in differentiation between
                             chondro-ectodermal   dysplasia   (Ellis–van
                             Creveld syndrome) and asphyxiating thoracic
                             dystrophy. Australas Radiol 16:401–410
                             Spranger S, Tariverdian G (1995). Symptomatic
                             heterozygosity in the Ellis–van Creveld syn-
                             drome? Clin Genet 47:217–220
                             Taylor GA, Jackman AL, Calvert AH, Harrup KR
                             (1984). Polycarpal and other abnormalities of
                             the wrist in chondroectodermal dysplasia: The
                             Ellis–van   Creveld   syndrome.   Radiology
                             151:393–396

Chromosomal Syndromes

Clinical features:

The common and well-recognised chromosomal disorders, i.e. Down, Klinefelter and Turner syndromes, have been mentioned elsewhere in this book. In addition, there are a number of rare cytogenetic conditions that enter into radiological differential diagnosis, especially during infancy. Trisomy 13 and 18, are the best known, but many others including Trisomy 8 may be encountered. Their features are protean and inconsistent but the possibility of a chromosomal abnormality arises in any unusual multiple malformation syndrome.

References:

Beighton P, Kozlowski KS, Gardner J, Smart R (1999). Broad clavicles in trisomy 8 mosaicism: a new sign. Skeletal Radiol 28:359–361

James AE (1971). Radiological features of most common chromosomal disorders. Clin Radiol 22:417–424

Kozlowski K, Collis J, Suter M, Sillence D (1988). The rib gap anomaly in partial or mosaic trisomy 8. Skeletal Radiol 17:251–254

Pilling DW, Levick RK (1978). Radiological abnormalities associated with the short arm of chromosome 9. Pediatr Radiol 6:215–221

Cleidocranial Dysplasia [119600]

Clinical features:

Large head, small face, increased mobility of shoulders, dental dysplasia, abnormal gait, hyper-mobility of joints, muscular hypotonia.

Radiographic features:

Defective skull ossification with wide sutures, wormian bones, large fontanelles, hypoplasia of the clavicles, retarded ossification of the pelvis and hands, pseudoepiphyses at the metacarpals and metatarsals.

Genetics:

AD; AR (rare, severe form).

Other considerations:

Cleidocranial dysplasia is often clinically innocuous and may merge with normality. It is probable that many affected persons remain un-diagnosed. A rare AR form characterised by

micrognathia, absent thumbs and digital apha-
langia is known as the Yunis–Varon syndrome
[216340].

References:

Ades LC, Morris LL, Richardson M, Pearson C,
Haan EA (1993). Congenital heart malfor-
mation in Yunis–Varon syndrome. J Med
Genet 30:788–792

Jarvis LJ, Keats TE (1974). Cleidocranial dysplasia: a review of 40 cases. Am J Roentgenol
121:5–11

Mundlos S (1999). Cleidocranial dysplasia: clinical and molecular genetics. J Med Gen-
et:36:177–182

Cloverleaf Skull (Kleeblattschädel Syndrome) [148800]

Clinical features:

The skull has a trilobular shape due to craniostenosis involving the coronal or lamboidal
sutures. Elbow ankylosis has been present in a
few instances.

Radiographic features:

Abnormal skull configuration with sutural synostosis.

Genetics:

Heterogeneous, usually non-genetic.

Other considerations:

The cloverleaf skull can occur as part of several
genetic syndromes, notably thanatophoric dysplasia and campomelic dysplasia.

References:

Angle B, Hersh JH, Christensen KM (1998).
Molecularly proven hypochondroplasia with
cloverleaf skull deformity: a novel association.
Clin Genet 54:417–420

Kozlowski K, Warren PS, Fisher CC (1985).
Cloverleaf skull with generalised bone dysplasia. Pediatr Radiol 15:412–414

Kozlowski K, Jequier S, Sillence D, Moir DH
(1987). Cloverleaf skull and bone dysplasias:
report of 4 cases. Australas Radiol 31:309–314

Warman ML, Mulliken JB, Hayward PG, Muller U
(1993). Newly recognised autosomal dominant
disorder with craniosynostosis. Am J Med
Genet 46:444–449

Cockayne Syndrome [216400]

Clinical features: Growth deficiency with mental retardation commencing in infancy, peculiar facies, photosensitive skin.

Radiographic features: Slim tubular bones with wide metaphyses and relatively large epiphyses, coxa valga, ovoid vertebral bodies, cerebral calcifications.

Genetics: AR (heterogeneous?).

Other considerations: This condition is sometimes confused with progeria.

References: Czeizel AE, Marchalko M (1995). Cockayne syndrome type III with high intelligence. Clin Genet 48:331–333

Nance MA, Berry SA (1992). Cockayne syndrome: review of 140 cases. Am J Med Genet 42:68–84

Riggs W Jr, Seiberg J (1972). Cockayne's syndrome: roentgen findings. Am J Roentgenol 116:623–633

Coffin–Lowry Syndrome [303600]

Clinical features: Short stature, mental deficiency, coarse facies, stubby hypermobile digits, pectus carinatum.

Radiographic features: Scheuerman-like changes in the spine, hyperostosis frontalis interna with excessive development of the frontal sinuses.

Genetics: XL with variable minor manifestations in carrier females.

Other considerations: The Coffin–Siris syndrome is the same disorder; the dislocated radial heads and small patellae in this condition represent variable phenotypic manifestations.

References: Gilgenkrantz S, Mujica P, Gruet P, Tridon P, Schweitzer F, Nivelon-Chevallier A, Nivelon JL, Couillault G, David A, Verloes A, Lambotte C, Piussan C, Mathieu M (1988). Coffin–Lowry syndrome: a multicenter study. Clin Genet 34:230–245

Hartsfield JK Jr, Hall BD, Grix AW, Kousseff BG, Salazar JF, Haufe JK Jr (1993). Pleiotropy in Coffin–Lowry syndrome: sensorineural hearing deficit and premature tooth loss as early manifestations. Am J Med Genet 45:552–557

Hunter AGW, Partington MW, Evans JA (1982). The Coffin–Lowry syndrome: Experience from four centres. Clin Genet 21(5):321–335

Coffin–Siris Syndrome (see Coffin–Lowry Syndrome)

Complex Carbohydrate Metabolic Disorders (Dysostosis Multiplex Group)

This group of conditions comprises the mucopolysaccharidoses, mucolipidoses and other related inherited metabolic disorders.

Each of these autonomous entities presents a different clinical picture but dwarfism, a coarse facies and progressive organ infiltration are general features. The radiographic changes involve all skeletal components (dysostosis multiplex) but the specific manifestations vary from condition to condition. The underlying molecular defects and enzymatic abnormalities have been identified in the majority of these disorders and definitive diagnosis is dependent upon laboratory investigations.

Genetically, these disorders are all autosomal recessive traits, except for MPS II (Hunter syndrome), which is X-linked.

Wherever possible, the syndromic references that are quoted in this section pertain to articles in which radiographic features are reviewed. Accounts of the complex molecular basis of these disorders predominate in the recent literature and for the sake of brevitus these have not been included.

General References: Grossman J, Dorst JP (1973). The mucopolysaccharidoses and mucolipidoses. In: Progress in Pediatric Radiology, 4. Intrinsic diseases of bones. Karger, Basel pp 495–510

Jaeken J, Carchon M (1993). The carbohydrate deficient glycoprotein syndromes: an overview. J Inherit Metab Dis 16:813–820

Leroy JG, Wiesman U (1993). In: Connective Tissue and its Heritable Disorders, Royce & Steinmann eds. Wiley-Liss, New York, pp 613–639

Neufeld E, Muenzer J (1995). The mucopolysaccharidoses. In: The Metabolic and Molecular

Basis of Inherited Disease, 7th edn. McGraw-Hill, New York, pp 2465-2494

Spranger J (1987). Mini review: Inborn errors of complex carbohydrate metabolism. Am J Med Genet 28:489-499

Whitley CB (1993). In: McKusick's Inherited Disorders of Connective Tissue, 5th edn. Beighton P ed. Mosby Year Book, St Louis, MO, pp 367-500

Syndromic References:

Mucopolysaccharidoses

MPS I-H (Hurler syndrome) [252800]

Thomas SL, Childress MH, Quinton B (1985). Hypoplasia of the odontoid with atlanto-axial subluxation in Hurler's syndrome. Pediatr Radiol 15:353-354

MPS I-S (Scheie syndrome) [252800]

Scheie HG, Hambrick GW Jr, Barness LA (1962). A newly recognised forme fruste of Hurler's disease (gargoylism). Am J Ophthalmol 53:753-769

MPS II (Hunter syndrome) [309900]

Young ID, Harper PS, Newcombe RG, Archer IM (1982). A clinical and genetic study of Hunter's syndrome. J Med Genet 19:408-411

MPS III type A-D (Sanfilippo syndrome) [252900, 252920, 252930, 252940]

Van de Kamp JJP, Niermeijer MF, von Figura K, Giesberts MA (1981). Genetic heterogeneity and clinical variability in the Sanfilippo syndrome (types A, B and C). Clin Genet 20:152-160

MPS IV type A and B (Morquio syndrome) [253000, 253010]

Langer LO Jr, Carey LS (1966). The roentgenographic features of the KS mucopolysaccharidosis of Morquio (Morquio-Brailsford's) disease. Am J Roentgenol 97:1-20

MPS VI (Maroteaux–Lamy syndrome) [253200]

> Strumpf DA, Austin JH, Crocker AC, Lafrance M
> (1973). Mucopolysaccharidosis type VI (Mar-
> oteaux–Lamy syndrome). Am J Dis Child
> 126:747–756

MPS VII (Sly syndrome) [253220]

> Sly WS, Quinton BA, McAlister WH, Rimoin DL
> (1973). Beta-glucuronidase deficiency: Report
> of clinical, radiologic and biochemical features
> of a new mucopolysaccharidosis. J Pediatr
> 82:249–255

Mucolipidoses

MLS I (Sialidosis) [256550]

> Spranger JW, Gehler J, Cantz M (1977). Mucoli-
> pidosis I, a sialidosis. Am J Med Genet 1:21–29

MLS II (Leroy I-cell disease) [252500]

> Lemaitre L, Remy J, Farriaux JP, Dhont JL,
> Walbaum R (1978). Radiological signs of
> mucolipidosis II or I-cell disease. A study of
> nine cases. Pediatr Radiol 7:97–105

MLS III (Pseudo-Hurler polydystrophy) [252600]

> Melhem R, Dorst JP, Scott CI Jr, McKusick VA
> (1973). Roentgen findings in mucolipidosis III
> (pseudo-Hurler polydystrophy). Radiology
> 106:153–160

Other Heteroglycanoses

Aspartylglycosaminuria [208400]

> Schmidt H, Ziegler R, Ullrich K, von Nengerke JH,
> Sewell AC. (1988). Skeletal changes in two
> German children with aspartylglycosaminuria.
> ROFO 149:143–146

Mannosidosis, alpha [248500], beta [248510]

> Spranger J, Gehler J, Cantz M (1976). The
> radiographic features of mannosidosis. Radi-
> ology 119:401–407

Galactosialidosis [2565400]

>Wenger DA, Tarby TJ, Wharton C (1978). Macular cherry-red spots and myoclonus with dementia: coexistent neuraminidase and beta-galactosidase deficiencies. Biochem Biophys Res Commun 82:589–595

Gangliosidosis, generalised GMI [230500]

>Van der Horst GTJ, Kleijer WJ, Hoogeveen AT, Huijmans JMG, Blom W, van Diggelen OP (1983). Morquio B syndrome: a primary defect in beta-galactosidase. Am J Med Genet 16:261–275

Fucosidosis [230000]

>Brill PW, Beratis NG, Kouseff G, Hirschhorn K (1975). Roentgenographic findings in fucosidosis type 2. Am J Roentgenol 124:75–82

Carbohydrate-deficient glycoprotein syndrome type I [212065]

>Garel C, Baumann C, Besnard M, Ogier H, Jaeken J, Hassan M (1998). Carbohydrate-deficient glycoprotein syndrome type I: a new cause of dysostosis multiplex. Skeletal Radiol 27:43–45

Conradi–Hünermann Syndrome (see Chondrodysplasia Punctata)

Cornelia de Lange Syndrome [122470]

Clinical features: Short stature, mental retardation, microcephaly, characteristic facies, inconsistent anomalies of the extremities.

Radiographic features: Short proximally implanted thumbs, radial hypoplasia, hypoplastic first metacarpal.

Genetics: Minor chromosomal deletion (?). AD (?).

Other considerations: The syndrome is rare but well recognised. Limb defects are very variable.

References: Jackson L, Kline AD, Barr MA, Koch S (1993). De Lange syndrome: A clinical review of 310 individuals. Am J Med Genet 47:940–946

Manouvrier S, Espinasse M, Vaast P, Boute O, Farre I, Dupont F, Puech F, Gosselin B, Farriaux J-P (1996). Brachmann–de Lange syndrome: pre- and postnatal findings. Am J Med Genet 62:268–273

Moeschler B, Cunniff C, Graham JM (1993). Radiological features in Brachmann–de Lange syndrome. Am J Med Genet 47:1006–1013

Craniocarpotarsal Syndrome (Whistling Face) (see Freeman–Sheldon Syndrome)

Craniodiaphyseal Dysplasia [122860; 218300]

Clinical features:	Distorted face, cranial nerve palsies, small stature, sometimes mental retardation.
Radiographic features:	Severe sclerosis and hyperostosis of the skull, cortical sclerosis and widening of the ribs and tubular bones.
Genetics:	AD/AR (further heterogeneity).
Other considerations:	The great severity of the craniofacial involvement distinguishes craniodiaphyseal dysplasia from other similar disorders.
References:	Brueton LA, Winter RM (1990). Craniodiaphyseal dysplasia. J Med Genet 27:701–706

Macpherson RJ (1974). Cranio-diaphyseal dysplasia, a disease or group of diseases? J Can Assoc Radiol 25:2–8

Schaefer B, Stein S, Oshman D, Rennart O, Thurnau G, Wall J, Bodensteiner J, Brown O (1986). Dominantly inherited craniodiaphyseal dysplasia: a new craniotubular dysplasia. Clin Genet 30:381–391

Tucker AS, Klein L, Anthony GJ (1976). Cranio-diaphyseal dysplasia, evolution over a 5-year period. Skeletal Radiol 1:47–52

Craniofacial Dysostosis (see Crouzon Syndrome)

Craniofacial Dysostosis with Diaphyseal Hyperplasia (see Osteosclerosis – Stanescu Type)

Craniometaphyseal Dysplasia [123000; 218400]

Clinical features: Large asymmetrical mandible, paranasal bossing, sometimes facial palsy and deafness.

Radiographic features: Sclerosis of the calvarium and base of the skull. Moderate expansion of the metaphyses of the long bones, especially the lower femur, without alteration in density.

Genetics: AD (a rare AR form is much more severe).

Other considerations: There is semantic confusion between craniometaphyseal dysplasia and Pyle disease [265900] (qv) but these conditions are separate and distinct entities.

References: Beighton P, Hamersma H, Horan F (1979). Cranio-metaphyseal dysplasia, variation in expression in a large kindred. Clin Genet 15:252–258

Beighton P (1995). Craniometaphyseal dysplasia (CMD), autosomal dominant form. J Med Genet 32:370–374

Penchaszadeh VB, Gutierriz ER, Figeueroa EP (1980). Autosomal recessive craniometaphyseal dysplasia. A J Med Genet 5:43–55

Spiro PC, Hamersma H, Beighton P (1975). Radiology of the autosomal dominant form of cranio-metaphyseal dysplasia. S Afr Med J 49:839–845

Craniosynostosis with Radial Defects (Baller–Gerold Syndrome) [218600]

Clinical features: Craniostenosis leading to skull deformity, stunted stature, malformation of forearms and thumbs. Variable mental retardation, deafness and abnormalities of spine, pelvis, anus, urogenital systems and heart.

Radiographic features: Absence of cranial sutures, malformation of radial ray structures.

Genetics: AR? Chromosomes show premature centromere separation.

Other considerations: Rare. Syndromic identity is uncertain.

References: Boudreaux JM, Colon MA, Lorusso GD, Parro EA, Pelias MZ (1990). Baller–Gerold syndrome: an 11th case of craniosynostosis and radial aplasia. Am J Med Genet 37:447–450

Cohen MM Jr, Toriello HV (1996). Is there a Baller–Gerold syndrome? Am J Med Genet (Editorial) 61:63–64

Dallapiccola B, Zelante L, Mingarelli R, Pellegrino M, Bertozzi V (1992). Baller–Gerold syndrome: case report and clinical and radiological review. Am J Med Genet 42:365–368

Crouzon Syndrome (Craniofacial Dysostosis) [123500]

Clinical features: Craniostenosis, midfacial hypoplasia, relative mandibular prognathism and bulging eyes produce a "frog face" appearance.

Radiographic features: Premature fusion of cranial sutures, especially coronal and sagittal, with brachycephaly, shallow orbits.

Genetics: AD with very variable expression.

Other considerations: The Crouzon syndrome differs from the other acrocephaly disorders by virtue of normality of the digits. Severity of facial involvement is extremely variable.

References: Anderson PJ, Hall CM, Evans RD, Jones BM, Hayward RD (1997). Hand anomalies in Crouzon syndrome. Skeletal Radiol 26:113–115

Cohen MM (1975). An etiologic and nosologic overview of craniosynostosis syndromes. In: Malformation Syndromes, Bergsma D ed. Birth Defects: Original Article Series, vol XI, no 2

Mafee MF, Valvassori GE (1981). Radiology of the craniofacial anomalies. Otolaryngol Clin North Am 14:939–988

De Barsy Syndrome [219150]

Clinical features: Cutis laxa, corneal clouding, mental retardation, dwarfism evident at birth, potentially lethal.

Radiographic features: Sclerotic foci in the skeleton are an important diagnostic indicator.

Genetics: AR.

Other considerations: Rare.

References: Karnes PS, Shamban AT, Olsen Dr, Fazio MJ, Falk RE (1992). De Barsy syndrome: report of a case, literature review, and elastin gene expression studies of the skin. Am J Med Genet 42:29–34

Stanton RP, Rao N, Scott C (1994). Orthopaedic manifestations in the de Barsey syndrome. J Ped Orthop 14:60–62

Dentinogenesis Imperfecta [125490] [125500]

Clinical features: Opaque purple or brownish fragile teeth.

Radiographic features: Absence of pulp chambers. Wormian bones in the cranial sutures.

Genetics: AD (Heterogeneous).

Other considerations: The condition may occur in isolation or in association with osteogenesis imperfecta and a few other rare genetic syndromes.

References: Beighton P (1981). Familial dentinogenesis imperfecta, blue sclerae and wormian bones without fractures: Another type of osteogenesis imperfecta? J Med Genet 18(2):124–128

Levin LS, Leaf SH, Jelmini RJ, Rose JJ, Rosenbaum KN (1983). Dentinogenesis imperfecta in the Brandywine isolate (DI type III): clinical, radiologic, and scanning electron microscopic studies of the dentition. Oral Surg Oral Med Oral Path 56:267–274

Shields ED, Bixler D, El-Kafrawy AM (1973). A proposed classification for heritable human dentine defect with a description of a new entity. Arch Oral Bio 18:543–553

Desbuquois Syndrome [251450]

Clinical features:	Micromelic dwarfism, joint laxity and multiple dislocations; mental retardation and glaucoma sometimes occur.
Radiographic features:	Generalised chondrodystrophy with vertebral and metaphyseal changes. Carpo-tarsal ossification is advanced and supernumerary ossification centres are present in the digits.
Genetics:	AR.
Other considerations:	Desbuquois syndrome must be distinguished from the Larsen syndrome [150250; 245600] and SEMDJL [271640].
References:	Le Merrer M, Young ID, Stanescu V, Maroteaux P (1991). Desbuquois syndrome. Eur J Pediatr 150:793–796. Shohat M, Lachman R, Gruber HE, Hsia YE, Golbus MS, Witt DR, Bodell A, Bryke CR, Hogge WA, Rimoin DL (1994). Desbuquois syndrome: clinical, radiographic, and morphologic characterization. Am J Med Genet 52:9–18

Diaphyseal Aclasis (see Multiple Cartilaginous Exostoses)

Diaphyseal Dysplasia (Camurati–Engelmann Disease) [131300]

Clinical features:	Prepubertal muscular pain and weakness, "tubular" legs.
Radiographic features:	Sclerosis of the diaphyseal cortices of the long bones, variable involvement of the base of the skull.
Genetics:	AD with variable expression and occasional non-penetrance.
Other considerations:	The use of the term "Ribbing disease" has lead to nosological confusion with the Ribbing type of multiple epiphyseal dysplasia, a very different disorder. An AR form which is associated with anaemia has been proposed [231095].

References: Grey AC, Wallace R, Crone M (1996). Engel-
                              mann's disease: a 45 year follow-up. J Bone
                              Joint Surg 78B:488–491
                              Kaftori JK, Kleinhaus U, Naueh Y (1987).
                              Progressive diaphyseal dysplasia (Camurati–
                              Engelmann): Radiographic follow-up and CT
                              findings. Radiology 164:777–782
                              Seeger LL, Hewel KC, Yao L, Gold RH, Mirra JM,
                              Chandnani VP, Eckardt JJ (1996). Ribbing
                              disease (multiple diaphyseal sclerosis): imaging
                              and differential diagnosis. Am J Roentgen
                              167:689–694

Diastrophic Dysplasia [222600]

Clinical features: Severe dwarfism with limb distortion, spinal
                              malalignment, cleft palate, rigid talipes equino-
                              varus, "hitchhiker" thumbs and irregular pinnae
                              of the ears.

Radiographic features: Shortened, undermodelled tubular bones, ovoid
                              first metacarpals, cone-shaped epiphyses of the
                              short tubular bones, delta deformity of the wrists,
                              accessory carpal ossification centres, flattened
                              epiphyses, delayed appearance of capital femoral
                              epiphyses, progressive kyphoscoliosis, equino-
                              varus deformity of the feet, interpedicular nar-
                              rowing in the lumbar spine.

Genetics: AR.

Other considerations: Diastrophic dysplasia usually causes very severe
                              dwarfing and disability. The condition, which
                              reaches a high frequency in Finland, is now
                              classified with atelosteogenesis II [256050] and
                              achondrogenesis IB [600972] as a defect of
                              sulphate transportation.

References: Hall BD (1996). Diastrophic dysplasia: extreme
                              variability within a sibship. Am J Med Genet
                              63:28–33
                              Hastbacka J, Superti-Furga A, Wilcox WR,
                              Rimoin DL, Cohn DH, Lander ES (1996).
                              Atelosteogenesis type II is caused by mutations
                              in the diastrophic dysplasia sulfate-transporter
                              gene (DTDST): evidence for a phenotypic series

involving three chondrodysplasias. Am J Hum Genet 58:255–262

Superti-Furga A, Rossi A, Steinmann B, Gitzelmann R (1996). A chondrodysplasia family produced by mutations in the diastrophic dysplasia sulfate transporter gene: genotype/phenotype correlations. Am J Med Genet 63:144–147

Distal Osteosclerosis [126250]

Clinical features: Clinically innocuous.

Radiographic features: Hyperostosis of the bones of the forearms and lower legs, together with mild cranial sclerosis.

Genetics: AD.

Other considerations: Encountered in several members of a South African family. Enters into the differential diagnosis of osteopetrosis and other sclerosing bone dysplasias.

References: Beighton P, Macrae M, Kozlowski K (1980). Distal osteosclerosis. Clin Genet 18:298–304

Distichiasis-Lymphedema Syndrome [153400]

Clinical features: Webbed neck, double row of eyelids, spinal extradural cysts, late-onset lymphedema of the lower limbs.

Radiographic features: Vertebral anomalies: enlarged interpedicular spaces, thinning of the pedicles, widening of the spinal canal with concavity of the dorsal surfaces of the vertebral bodies.

Genetics: AD.

Other considerations: The epidural cysts, if present, may cause serious neurological dysfunction.

References: Dale RF (1987). Primary lymphedema when found with distichiasis is of the type defined as bilateral hyperplasia by lymphography. J Med Genet 24:170–171

Kolin T, Johns KJ, Wadlington WB, Butler MG, Sunalp MA, Wright KW (1991). Hereditary lymphedema and distichiasis. Arch Ophthal 109:980–981

Down Syndrome (Trisomy 21) [190685]

Clinical features: Mental retardation, stunted stature, flat occiput, "mongoloid" facies, simian crease, congenital cardiac defects.

Radiographic features: Brachycephaly, flared ilia with reduced acetabular angles and iliac indices, stubby digits, clinomicrodactyly of fifth fingers.

Genetics: Trisomy of chromosome 21. Infrequently translocation or mosaicism.

Other considerations: Down syndrome is the most common and best recognised mental deficiency syndrome, the prevalence in neonates being about 1 in 600. Radiology may be helpful but diagnosis is confirmed by cytogenetic studies.

References: Miller JD, Grace MG, Lampard R (1986). Computed tomography of the upper cervical spine in Down syndrome. J Comput Assist Tomogr 10:589–592

Pueschel SM, Scola FH (1987). Atlantoaxial instability in individuals with Down syndrome: Epidemiologic, radiographic and clinical studies. Pediatrics 80:555–560

Taybi H, Kane P (1968). Small acetabular and iliac angles and associated diseases. Radiol Clin North Am 6:215–220

Dyggve–Melchior–Clausen Dysplasia [223800]

Clinical features: Short-limb dwarfism, crouching stance, mental retardation.

Radiographic features: Generalised platyspondyly with a characteristic shape of the vertebral bodies, crenated iliac crests, medial elongation of the femoral necks, generalised involvement of the metaphyses and epiphyses.

Genetics: AR.

Other considerations:	The Smith–McCort syndrome has identical features, with the exception of normal mentality.
References:	Beighton P (1990). Dyggve–Melchior–Clausen syndrome. J Med Genet 27:512–515
	Spranger J, Maroteaux P, Der Kaloustian VM (1975). The Dyggve–Melchior–Clausen syndrome. Radiology 114:415–422
	Winship WS, Rubin DL (1992). The Dyggve–Melchior–Clausen syndrome in Indian siblings. Clin Genet 42:240–245

Dyschondrosteosis [127300]

Clinical features:	Mild shortening of stature, Madelung deformity of the wrists.
Radiographic features:	Shortened radius with lateral bowing and oblique distal articular surface. Dorsal subluxation of the distal ulna. The tibia and fibula are shortened but have a normal configuration.
Genetics:	AD (rare AR form with additional shortening of hands and feet).
Other considerations:	A Madelung deformity is often the presenting feature but mild cases may be asymptomatic and remain undiagnosed.
References:	Dawe C, Wynne-Davis R, Fulford GE (1982). Clinical variation in dyschondrosteosis: a report on 13 individuals in 8 families. J Bone Joint Surg [Br] 64:377–381
	Langer LO Jr (1965). Dyschondrosteosis: A heritable bone dysplasia with characteristic roentgenographic features. Am J Roentgenol 95:178–188

Dysosteosclerosis [224300]

Clinical features:	Small stature, fractures, dental anomalies.
Radiographic features:	Generalised osteosclerosis with platyspondyly, flared osteoporotic metaphyses and sclerotic epiphyses.
Genetics:	AR.

Other considerations: Less than 20 patients, all children, have been described. Heterogeneity is possible.

References: Chitayat D, Silver K, Azouz EM (1992). Skeletal dysplasia, intracerebral calcifications, optic atrophy, hearing impairment and mental retardation: Nosology of dysosteosclerosis. Am J Med Genet 43:517–523

                           Houston CS, Gerrard JW, Ives EJ (1978). Dysosteosclerosis. Am J Radiol 130:988–996

Dysostosis Multiplex Congenita (see Complex Carbohydrate Disorders)

Dysplasia Epiphysealis Hemimelica (Trevor Disease) [127800]

Clinical features: Unilateral swelling and deformity of the knee and ankle, onset usually in childhood.

Radiographic features: Asymmetrical irregular overgrowth and calcification of one or more epiphyses and tarsal bones.

Genetics: Usually non-genetic.

Other considerations: The localisation of the changes to one side of a limb is an important diagnostic indicator. In an uncommon AD form, osteochondromata represent an additional feature.

References: Azouz EM, Slomic AM, Marton D, Rigault P, Finidori G (1985). The variable manifestations of dysplasia epiphysealis hemimelica. Pediatr Radiol 15:44–49

                           Connor JM, Horan FT, Beighton P (1983). Dysplasia epiphysealis hemimelica. J Bone Jt Surg [Br] 65:350–354

                           Greenspan A, Steiner G, Sotelo D, Norman A, Sotelo A, Sotelo-Ortiz F (1986). Mixed sclerosing bone dysplasia coexisting with dysplasia epiphysealis hemimelica (Trevor-Fairbank disease). Skeletal Radiol 15:452–454

                           Lang IM, Azouz EM (1997). MRI appearances of dysplasia epiphysealis hemimelica of the knee. Skeletal Radiol 26:226–229

Dyssegmental Dysplasia [224400; 224410]

Clinical features: Lethal dwarfism with short bowed limbs.

Radiographic features: Malsegmentation of the spine, coronal cleft vertebrae, short broad bowed tubular bones, short ribs, accentuated carpal bone maturation.

Genetics: AR.

Other considerations: Very rare. Silverman–Handmaker and Rolland–Desbuquois types are recognised.

References: Aleck KA, Grix A, Clericuzio C, Kaplan P, Adomian GE, Lachman R, Rimoin DL (1987). Dyssegmental dysplasias: clinical, radiographic and morphologic evidence of heterogeneity. Am J Med Genet 27:295–312

Fasanelli S, Kozlowski K, Reiter S, Sillence D (1985). Dyssegmental dysplasia. Skel Radiol 14:173–177

Maroteaux P, Manouvrier S, Bonaventure J, Le Merrer M (1996). Dyssegmental dysplasia with glaucoma. Am J Med Genet 63:46–49

EEC Syndrome (Ectrodactyly, Ectodermal Dysplasia, Facial Clefts) [129900]

Clinical features: Variable split hand or foot with cleft lip or palate, dental, hair and skin involvement and dysplasia of the lacrimal puncti or ducts. Urinary tract malformations are sometimes present.

Radiographic features: Variable absence, fusion and hypoplasia of the digits.

Genetics: AD with variable expression.

Other considerations: There is considerable nosological confusion with the Adams-Oliver syndrome [100300] and the Split-hand Split-foot Malformation (SHFM) [183600].

References: Buss PW, Hughes HE, Clarke A (1995). Twenty-four cases of the EEC syndrome: clinical presentation and management. J Med Genet 32:716–723

Rodini ESO, Richieri-Costa A (1990). EEC syndrome: report on 20 new patients, clinical and genetic considerations. Am J Med Genet 37:42–53

Roelfsema NM, Cobben JM (1996). The EEC syndrome: a literature study. Clin Dysmorph 5:115–127

Ehlers–Danlos Syndrome [130000; 130090]

Clinical features: Joint hypermobility, dermal hyperextensibility, tissue fragility leading to cutaneous scarring.

Radiographic features: Sequelae of articular laxity – subluxed or dislocated joints, spinal malalignment. Multiple small subcutaneous calcified spheroids may be present over the shafts of the long bones and mimic phleboliths or parasites.

Genetics: Very heterogeneous, AD (most forms), XL and AR types are rare.

Other considerations: The syndrome is relatively common, reaching a minimum prevalence in Britain of 1 in 150,000. At least 11 different varieties have been delineated but the autosomal dominant types I, II and III account for more than 90% of all patients. The continuing elucidation of the molecular defects is resulting in amendments to the nosology of the EDS.

References:
Beighton P (1970). The Ehlers–Danlos syndrome. Heinemann, London

Beighton P, Thomas M (1969). Radiological aspects of the Ehlers–Danlos syndrome. Clin Radiol 20:354–360

Hagino H, Eda I, Takashima S, Takeshita K, Sugitani A (1985). Computed tomography in patients with Ehlers–Danlos syndrome. Neuroradiology 27:443–445

Ellis–Van Creveld Syndrome (see Chrondroectodermal Dysplasia)

Enchondromatosis (Ollier Disease) [166000]

Clinical features: Protuberances and asymmetry of the digits and less commonly other regions. Fractures through affected areas.

Radiographic features: Irregular radiolucent areas in the metaphyses and later the diaphyses of tubular bones and occasionally the flat bones.

Genetics: Non-genetic?

Other considerations: Enchondral changes are also a component of a few rare inherited syndromes, notably metachondromatosis and spondyloenchondrodysplasia [271550].

References: Feldman F (1974). Cartilaginous lesions of the bones and soft tissues: a critical view. Clin Radiol 4:477–482

Mainzer F, Minagi H, Steinbach HL (1971). The variable manifestations of multiple enchondromatosis. Radiology 99:377–388

Spranger J, Kemperdieck H, Bakowski H, Opitz JM (1978). Two peculiar types of enchondromatosis. Pediatr Radiol 7:215–219

Enchondromatosis with Haemangioma (Maffucci Syndrome) [166000]

Clinical features: Digital and limb irregularity and deformity due to multiple enchondromata and haemangiomata. Tendency to malignant degeneration.

Radiographic features: Multiple enchondromata with severe bone deformities, radiolucent haemangiomata which often contain phleboliths.

Genetics: Non-genetic?

Other considerations: The Maffucci syndrome must be distinguished from the Klippel–Trenaunay–Weber syndrome [149000], in which angiomatous changes are associated with bone hypertrophy, but not with enchondromata. Genochondromatosis is a sub-category [137360].

References:

Hisaoka M, Aoki T, Kouho H, Chosa H, Hashimoto H (1997). Maffucci's syndrome associated with spindle cell hemangioendothelioma. Skeletal Radiol 26:191–194

Kaplan RP, Wang JT, Amron DM, Kaplan L (1994). Maffucci's syndrome: two case reports with a literature review. J Am Acad Derm 29:894–899

Loewinger RJ, Lichtenstein JR, Dodson WE, Eisen AZ (1977). Maffucci's syndrome: a mesenchymal dysplasia and multiple tumour syndrome. Br J Derm 96:317–322

Endosteal Hyperostosis, van Buchem Form [239100]

Clinical features: Mandibular overgrowth and asymmetry, variable facial nerve paralysis and deafness.

Radiographic features: Severe sclerosis and hyperostosis of the calvarium, base of the skull and mandible. Generalised sclerosis in the cortices of the long bones.

Genetics: AR.

Other considerations: About 20 patients have been identified, the majority in The Netherlands, with aggregation in an inbred community on the island of Urk.

References:

Dixon JM, Cull RE, Gamble P (1982). Two cases of van Buchem's disease. J Neurol Neurosurg Psychiatry 45:913–918

Eastman JR, Bixley D (1977). Generalised cortical hyperostosis (van Buchem disease). Nosological considerations. Radiology 125:297–303

Endosteal Hyperostosis, Worth Form [144750]

Clinical features: Mild mandibular overgrowth with occasional facial palsy.

Radiographic features: Mild to moderate sclerosis of the calvarium and base of the skull, generalised skeletal sclerosis, especially in the diaphyseal cortices of the tubular bones.

Genetics: AD.

Other considerations: This disorder is very similar to the benign or tarda form of osteopetrosis. It is the subject of semantic confusion with endosteal hyperostosis, van Buchem form [239100], which is much more severe. Endosteal hyperostosis with cerebellar hypoplasia is a rare autonomous disorder that is inherited as an AR trait [213002].

References: Ades LC, Morris LL, Burns R, Haan EA (1994). Neurological involvement in Worth type endosteal hyperostosis: report of a family. Am J Med Genet 51:46–50

Charrow J, Poznanski AK, Unger FM, Robinow M (1991). Autosomal recessive cerebellar hypoplasia and endosteal hyperostosis. Am J Med Genet 41:464–468

Gorlin RJ, Glass L (1977). Autosomal dominant osteosclerosis. Radiology 125:547

Engelmann Disease (see Diaphyseal Dysplasia)

Faciogenital Dysplasia (see Aarskog Syndrome)

Familial Articular Hypermobility [147900]

Clinical features: Articular hypermobility with a propensity to multiple dislocations. Spinal malalignment and foot deformity may occur.

Radiographic features: Dislocations and subluxations.

Genetics: AD (heterogeneous), AR form?

Other considerations: The familial articular hypermobility syndromes may be innocuous or lead to considerable disability. Distinction from Ehlers–Danlos syndrome type III may be difficult.

References: Beighton P, Horan F (1970). Dominant inheritance of generalised articular hypermobility. J Bone Joint Surg [Br] 52(1):145–151

Grahame R (1999). Joint hypermobility and genetic collagen disorders: are they related? Arch Dis Child 80(2):188–191

Fanconi Pancytopenia Syndrome [227650]

Clinical features:	Short stature, hypoplasia of thumbs and forearms, pancytopenia, dermal pigmentation.
Radiographic features:	Variable radial ray hypoplasia (thumb, radius).
Genetics:	AR.
Other considerations:	Leukaemia is sometimes a late complication.
References:	Duckworth-Rysiecki G, Hulten M, Mann J, Taylor AMR (1984). Clinical and cytogenetic diversity in Fanconi's anaemia. J Med Genet 21:197
	Giampietro PF, Adler-Brecher B, Verlander PC, Pavlakis SG, Davis JG, Auerbach AD (1993). The need for more accurate and timely diagnosis in Fanconi anemia: a report from the International Fanconi Anemia Registry. Pediatrics 91:116–1120
	Juhl JH, Wesenberg RL, Gwinn JL (1967). Roentgenographic findings in Fanconi's anaemia. Radiology 89:846–653

Femoral Facial Syndrome (Proximal Focal Femoral Dysplasia) [134780]

Clinical features:	Severe femoral hypoplasia, variable skeletal anomalies in the extremities, characteristic facies.
Radiographic features:	Proximal focal femoral dysgenesis, which may be asymmetrical. Inconsistent hypoplasia and synostoses in the limb bones.
Genetics:	AD? Non-genetic.
Other considerations:	Unilateral focal femoral dysplasia is fairly common and non-genetic. The association of bilateral femoral hypoplasia and an unusual facies has been recognised but there is controversy concerning the syndromic status of this combination.

References:

Lord J, Beighton P (1981). The femoral hypoplasia – unusual facies syndrome: a genetic entity? Clin Genet 20:267–275

Robinow M, Sonek J, Buttino L, Veghte A (1995). Femoral-facial syndrome – prenatal diagnosis – autosomal dominant inheritance. Am J Med Genet 57:397–399

Sabry MA, Obenbergerova D, Al-Sawan R, Al Saleh Q, Farah S, Al-Awadi SA, Farag TI (1996). Femoral hypoplasia-unusual facies syndrome with bifid hallux, absent tibia, and macrophallus: a report of a Bedouin baby. J Med Genet 33:165–167

Fibrochondrogenesis [228520]

Clinical features: Lethal neonatal dwarfism.

Radiographic features: Widening of the metaphyses, pear-shaped vertebral bodies, coronal fissure of the vertebral bodies.

Genetics: AR.

Other considerations: Very rare.

References:

Eteson DJ, Adonian GE, Ornoyu A, Koide T, Sugiura Y, Calabro A, Lungarotti S, Mastroiacovo P, Lachman RS, Rimoin DL (1984). Fibrochondrogenesis: Radiologic and histologic studies. Am J Med Genet 19:277–290

Martinez-Frias ML, Garcia A, Cuevas J, Rodriguez JI, Urioste M (1996). A new case of fibrochondrogenesis from Spain. J Med Genet 33:429–431

Whitley CB, Langer LO Jr, Ophoven J, Gilbert EF, Gonzalez CH, Mammel M, Coleman M, Rosemberg S, Rodriques CJ, Sibley R, Horton WA, Opitz JM, Gorlin RJ (1984). Fibrochondrogenesis: lethal, autosomal recessive chondrodysplasia with distinctive cartilage histopathology. Am J Med Genet 19:265–275

Fibrodysplasia Ossificans Progressiva [135100]

Clinical features: Painful swellings, usually on the trunk, with subsequent ossification in connective tissues, leading to widespread rigidity and profound disability.

Radiographic features: In early stages ill-defined opacities near tendon insertions simulate exostoses. Later widespread subcutaneous ossification is evident. Hypoplasia of the first fingers and toes is a variable feature.

Genetics: AD.

Other considerations: The condition is rare but well defined, with a prevalence of about one per million. Most affected persons represent new gene mutations and a paternal age effect has been demonstrated.

References: Cremin B, Connor JM, Beighton P (1982). The radiological spectrum of fibrodysplasia ossificans progressiva. Clin Radiol 33:499–508

Connor JM, Evans DAP (1982). Fibrodysplasia ossificans progressiva: the clinical features and natural history of 34 patients. J Bone Joint Surg 64:76–83

Connor JM, Skirton H, Lunt PW (1993). A three generation family with fibrodysplasia ossificans progressiva. J Med Genet 30:687–689

Smith R, Athanasou NA, Vipond SE (1996). Fibrodysplasia (myositis) ossificans progressiva: clinicopathological features and natural history. Quart J Med 89:445–456

Fibrous Dysplasia (Jaffe–Lichtenstein Syndrome) [174800]

Clinical features: Deformity, pain and fractures of long bones, cutaneous pigmented café-au-lait macules.

Radiographic features: Mixed lytic and sclerotic lesions that produce a "ground-glass" appearance and lead to deformities and fractures of the long bones. The changes may be monostotic.

Genetics: Usually non-genetic. Rare AD form.

Other considerations: The monostotic type is fairly common and is often only recognised on an incidental radiograph. There are a few reports of a symmetrical autosomal dominant form.

References: Grabias SL, Campbell CJ (1977). Fibrous dysplasia. Clin Orthop 8:771–776

Taconis WK (1988). Osteosarcoma in fibrous dysplasia. Skeletal Radiol 17:163–170

Viljoen DL, Versfeld GA, Losken W, Beighton P (1988). Polyostotic fibrous dysplasia with cranial hyperostosis: new entity or severe form of polyostotic fibrous dysplasia? Am J Med Genet 29:661–667

Fibrous Dysplasia of the Jaws (see Cherubism)

Fibrous Dysplasia with Pigmentary Skin Changes and Precocious Puberty (McCune–Albright Syndrome) [174800]

Clinical features: Short stature, variable skeletal deformity, café-aulait macules, precocious puberty in girls. Endocrine disturbance and malignancy often develop.

Radiographic features: Radiolucent "ground-glass" regions of fibrosis, especially in the long bones, advanced skeletal age.

Genetics: Non-genetic.

Other considerations: The McCune–Albright syndrome is rare and only about 3% of persons with polyostotic fibrous dysplasia have the former condition. Albright hereditary osteodystrophy (pseudohypoparathyroidism) is a different disorder [103580].

References: Chanson P, Dib A, Visot A, Derome PJ (1994). McCune–Albright syndrome and acromegaly: clinical studies and responses to treatment in five cases. Europ J Endocr 131:229–234

Happle R (1986). The McCune–Albright syndrome: a lethal gene surviving by mosaicism. Clin Genet 29:321–324

Majzoub JA, Scully RE (1993). A six-year old boy with multiple bone lesions, repeated fractures, and sexual precocity. New Eng J Med 328:496–502

Tinschert S, Gerl H, Gewies A, Jung H-P, Nürnberg P (1999). McCune–Albright syndrome: clinical and molecular evidence of mosaicism in an unusual giant patient. Am J Med Genet 83:100–108

Fibrous Dysplasia, Congenital Generalised Form (Myofibromatosis) [228550]

Clinical features:	Multiple fibromatosis lesions in the bones, skin, muscles and internal organs; present in infancy; prognosis poor.
Radiographic features:	Multiple cystic abnormalities in the metaphyses and diaphyses.
Genetics:	AR.
Other considerations:	Radiographic changes resemble those of enchondromatosis.
References:	Baer JW, Radkowski MA (1973). Congenital multiple fibromatosis: a case report with review of the world literature. Am J Roentgen 118:200–205
	Evans GA, Park WM (1978). Familial multiple non-osteogenic fibromata. J Bone Joint Surg [Br] 60:416–419
	Modi N (1982). Congenital generalized fibromatosis. Arch Dis Child 57:881–882.

Focal Dermal Hypoplasia (see Goltz Syndrome)

Foetal Alcohol Syndrome

Clinical features:	Low birth weight, microcephaly, mental retardation, typical facies with blepharophimosis and absent nasolabial folds.
Radiographic features:	Occasionally radio-ulnar synostosis with fusions in the tarsus and carpus, punctate epiphyses and small terminal phalanges.
Genetics:	Non-genetic. Foetal damage results from maternal alcohol ingestion.

Other considerations: Prevalence unknown, may be fairly common, severity is very variable and mild cases merge into normality.

References:
Cremin BJ, Jaffer Z (1981). Radiological aspects of the foetal alcohol syndrome. Pediatr Radiol 11(3):151–153

Jaffer Z, Nelson M, Beighton P (1981). Bone fusion in the foetal alcohol syndrome. J Bone Joint Surg [Br] 638(4):569–571

Johnson VP, Swayze VW II, Sato Y, Andreasen NC (1996). Fetal alcohol syndrome: craniofacial and central nervous system manifestations. Am J Med Genet 61:329–339

Freeman–Sheldon Syndrome (Whistling Face Syndrome; Craniocarpotarsal Dystrophy) [193700]

Clinical features: Small pursed mouth, ulnar deviation of digits, inconsistent skeletal abnormalities.

Radiographic features: Retarded bone age.

Genetics: AD with very variable expression.

Other considerations: Diagnosis is essentially clinical. Reclassification as a form of distal arthrogryposis has been proposed.

References:
Bamshad M, Jorde LB, Carey JC (1996). A revised and extended classification of the distal arthrogryposes. Am J Med Genet 65:277–281

O'Connell DJ, Hall CM (1977). Cranio-carpotarsal dysplasia. A report of 7 cases. Radiology 123:719–723

Wang TR, Lin SJ (1987). Further evidence for genetic heterogeneity of whistling face or Freeman–Sheldon syndrome in a Chinese family. Am J Med Genet 28:471–475

Zampino G, Conti G, Balducci F, Moschini M, Macchiailo M, Mastroiacovo P (1996). Severe form of Freeman–Sheldon syndrome associated with brain anomalies and hearing loss. Am J Med Genet 62:293–296

Frontometaphyseal Dysplasia [305620]

Clinical features: Prominent supraorbital ridge, mandibular hypoplasia, dental abnormalities, long fingers.

Radiographic features: Pronounced sclerosis and overgrowth of the supraorbital ridges and progressive, patchy sclerosis of the calvarium are the major features. The skeleton shows widespread but mild dysplastic changes, with supra-acetabular constriction of the iliac bones and lack of modelling of the tubular bones of hands and feet.

Genetics: XL with partial manifestation in carrier females.

Other considerations: This condition may be the same entity as the Oto-palato-digital syndrome.

References: Beighton P, Hamersma H (1980). Frontometaphyseal dysplasia: autosomal dominant or X-linked? J Med Genet 17:53–56

Glass RBJ, Rosenbaum KN (1995). Frontometaphsyeal dysplasia: neonatal radiographic diagnosis. Am J Med Genet 57:1–5

Superti-Furga A, Gimelli F (1987). Fronto-metaphyseal dysplasia and the oto-palato-digital syndrome. Dysmorph Clin Genet 1:2–5

Fucosidosis (see Complex Carbohydrate Metabolic Disorders)

Fuhrmann Dysplasia

Clinical features: Short stature.

Radiographic features: Tall, narrow vertebrae are a diagnostic indicator. The ribs are slender and sloping. Coxa vara may be present.

Genetics: AD with variable expression (?).

Other considerations: Very rare. This condition is a different entity from Fuhrmann syndrome, in which fibular hypoplasia is associated with extreme femoral bowing and digital abnormalities. [228930].

References: Fuhrmann W, Nagele E, Guglar R Adili E (1972). Dwarfism with disproportionately high vertebral bodies. Humangenetik 16:271–282

Lipson AH, Kozlowski K, Barylak A, Marsden W (1991). Fuhrmann syndrome of right angle bowed femora, absence of fibulae and digital anomalies: two further cases. Am J Med Genet 41:176–179

Galactosialidoses (see Complex Carbohydrate Metabolic Disorders)

Gardner Syndrome (Familial Colonic Polyposis) [175100]

Clinical features:	Polyposis of the colon with malignant change in adulthood, epidermal cysts that do not become evident until late childhood.
Radiographic features:	Osteomata of the skull and jaws, delayed eruption of teeth.
Genetics:	AD.
Other considerations:	The Gardner syndrome is fairly common and, in view of the risk of neoplasia, early diagnosis is very important. Presymptomatic diagnosis using molecular linkage techniques is feasible in some affected families.
References:	Krush AJ, Traboulsi EI, Offerhaus GJA, Maumenee IH, Yardley JH, Levin LS (1988). Hepatoblastoma, pigmented ocular fundus lesions and jaw lesions in Gardner syndrome. Am J Med Genet 29:323–332
	Lynch HT (1996). Desmoid tumors: genotype-phenotype differences in familial adenomatous polyposis: a nosological dilemma. (Editorial) Am J Hum Genet 59:1184–1185
	Thakker N, Davies R, Horner K, Armstrong J, Clancy T, Guy S, Harris R, Sloan P, Evans G (1995). The dental phenotype in familial adenomatous polyposis: diagnostic application of a weighted scoring system for changes on dental panoramic radiographs. J Med Genet 32:458–464
	Utsunomiya J, Nakamura T (1975). The occult osteomatous changes in the mandible in patients with familial polyposis coli. Br J Surg 62:45–51

Gaucher Disease [230800]

Clinical features:

Adult chronic or non-neuropathic type (relatively common, predilection for Ashkenazi Jews): splenomegaly, dyshemopoiesis, collapse of femoral heads, pseudo-osteomyelitis. Fluctuating, slowly progressive course.

Infantile neuropathic type (rare, panethnic): death in infancy from cerebral involvement, hepatosplenomegaly.

Juvenile type (rare, mostly occurs in Scandinavia): predominant involvement of skeleton and basal ganglia.

Radiographic features:

Metaphyseal widening, especially of lower femur, coarse trabeculation and radiolucent cysts in the long bones, aseptic necrosis of femoral heads, occasional vertebral wedging.

Genetics:

AR (heterogeneous).

Other considerations:

The same enzyme, beta-glucosidase, is defective in all forms of Gaucher disease. Considerable intramolecular heterogeneity is present.

References:

Beighton P, Goldblatt J, Sacks S (1982). Bone involvement in Gaucher disease. In: Progress in Clinical and Biological Research, Desnick J ed. Alan Liss, New York, pp 95–106

Goldblatt J, Sacks S, Dall D, Beighton P (1988). Total hip arthroplasty in Gaucher's disease: long-term prognosis. Clin Orthop 228:94–98

Hermann G, Pastores GM, Abdelwahib IF, Lorberboym AM (1997). Gaucher disease: assessment of skeletal involvement and therapeutic responses to enzyme replacement. Skeletal Radiol 26:687–696

Myers HS, Cremin B, Beighton P Sacks S (1975). Chronic Gaucher disease; radiological findings in 17 South African cases. Br J Radiol 48:465–471

Wasserstein MP, Martignetti JA, Zeitlin R, Lumerman H, Solomon M, Grace ME, Desnick RJ (1999). Type I Gaucher disease presenting with extensive mandibular lytic lesions: identification and expression of a novel acid β-

Glucosidase mutation. Am J Med Genet 84:334–339

Geleophysic Dysplasia [231050]

Clinical features: Stunted stature, joint contractures, "happy" facies, cardiac failure, hepatosplenomegaly.

Radiographic features: Mesomelia, short phalanges, J-shaped sella turcica.

Genetics: AR.

Other considerations: Rare.

References: Pontz BF, Stoss H, Jenschke F, Freisinger P, Karbowski A, Spranger J (1996). Clinical and ultrastructural findings in three patients with geliophysic dysplasia. Am J Med Genet 63:50–54

Rosser EM, Wilkinson AR, Hurst JA, McGaughran JM, Donnai D (1995). Geleophysic dysplasia: a report of three affected boys – prenatal ultrasound does not detect recurrence. Am J Med Genet 58:217–221

Shohat M, Gruber HE, Pagon RA, Witcoff LJ, Lachman R, Ferry D, Flaum E, Rimoin DL (1990). Geleophysic dysplasia: a storage disorder affecting the skin, bone, liver, heart and trachea. J Pediat 117:227–232

Geroderma Osteodysplastica [231070]

Clinical features: Short stature, premature facial ageing, atrophy and hyperlaxity of the skin on back of hands and feet, articular hypermobility, susceptibility to fractures.

Radiographic features: Osteoporosis of spine, generalised platyspondyly, hip dislocation or subluxation. A peg-shaped metaphyseal indentation into the epiphyses, especially at the knees, may represent a specific radiological feature in early childhood.

Genetics: AR.

Other Considerations: There is clinical overlap with the De Barsy syndrome [219150] and cutis laxa with bone dystrophy [219200].

References:

Al-Torki NA, Al-Awadi SA, Cindro-Heberie L, Sabry MA (1997). Gerodermia osteodysplastica in a Bedoiun sibship: further delineation of the syndrome. Clin Dysmorph 6:51–55

Eich GF, Steinmann B, Hodler J, Exner GU, Giedion A (1996). Metaphyseal peg in geroderma osteodysplasticum: a new genetic bone marker and a specific finding? Am J Med Genet 63:62–67

Hunter AGW (1988). Is geroderma osteodysplastica underdiagnosed? J Med Genet 25:854–857

Lisker R, Hernandez A, Martinez-Lavin M, Muchinick O, Armas C, Reyes P, Robles-Gil J (1979). Gerodermia osteodysplastica hereditaria: report of three affected brothers and literature review. Am J Med Genet 3:389–395

Giedion–Langer Syndrome (see Trichorhinophalangeal Dysplasia or Acrodysplasia with Exostoses)

GMI Gangliosidosis (see Complex Carbohydrate Metabolic Disorders)

Goldenhar Syndrome (Oculoauriculo-vertebral Dysplasia) [164210]

Clinical features: Unilateral mandibular hypoplasia in association with ocular colobomata plus auricular and vertebral abnormalities.

Radiographic features: Mandibular hypoplasia. Vertebral fusions, hemivertebrae, supernumerary vertebrae.

Genetics: Uncertain, possibly multifactorial.

Other considerations: There are many reports in the literature. Syndromic boundaries are ill defined and partial cases are not uncommon. A common pathogenesis with the CHARGE association [214800] has been proposed.

References: Boles DJ, Bodurtha J, Nance WE (1987). Gold-
                        enhar complex in discordant monozygotic
                        twins: a case report and review of the literature.
                        Am J Med Genet 28:103–109
                        Rollnick BR, Kaye CI, Nagatoshi K, Hauck W,
                        Martin AO (1987). Oculoauriculovertebral dys-
                        plasia and variants: phenotypic characteristics
                        of 294 patients. Am J Med Genet 26:361–375
                        Stoll C, Viville B, Treisser A, Gasser B (1998). A
                        family with dominant oculoauriculovertebral
                        spectrum. Am J Med Genet 78:345–349
                        Van Meter TD, Weaver DD (1996). Oculo-
                        auriculo-vertebral spectrum and the CHARGE
                        association: clinical evidence for a common
                        pathogenetic mechanism. Clin Dysmorph
                        5:187–196

Goltz Syndrome (Focal Dermal Hypoplasia) [305600]

Clinical features: Linear areas of dermal hypoplasia. Dystrophic
                        nails, hypoplastic teeth, ocular changes, variable
                        skeletal malformations, digital anomalies, fre-
                        quent mental retardation.

Radiographic features: Variable but widespread anomalies, including
                        clavicular hypoplasia, scoliosis, spina bifida,
                        non-specific changes in the hands and ribs,
                        failure of pelvic bone fusion, osteoporosis, linear
                        striations in the tubular bones.

Genetics: X-linked dominant; lethal in males.

Other considerations: The variability of the clinical and radiographic
                        manifestations is noteworthy.

References: Bellosta M, Trespiolli D, Ghiselli E, Capra E,
                        Scappaticci S (1996). Focal dermal hypoplasia:
                        report of a family with 7 affected women in 3
                        generations. Eur J Dermatol 6:499–500
                        Goltz RW (1992). Focal dermal hypoplasia
                        syndrome: an update. (Editorial) Arch Derm
                        128:1108–1111
                        Knockaert D, Dequeker J (1979). Osteopathia
                        striata and focal dermal hypoplasia. Skeletal
                        Radiol 4:223–227

Gorham Osteolysis (see Osteolysis Syndromes)

Grebe Dysplasia [200700]

Clinical features:	Dwarfism with gross limb shortening, variable polydactyly and small misshapen digits. The head and trunk are normal and life span is unimpaired.
Radiographic features:	Diaphyseal shortening of the limb bones, marked digital hypoplasia, skull and spine are normal.
Genetics:	AR. Large affected families in Brazil and China.
Other considerations:	Grebe dysplasia was formerly known as Achondrogenesis type II. In the revised nosology this designation is reserved for a severe form of short-limbed dwarfism which is lethal in the neonatal period [200610].
References:	Garcia-Castro (1975). Non-lethal achondrogenesis (Grebe-Quelce-Salgado type) in two Puerto Rico sibships. J Pediat 87:948–952
	Kumar D, Curtis D, Blank CE (1984). Grebe chondrodysplasia and brachydactyly in a family. Clin Genet 25:68–72

Hajdu–Cheney Syndrome (see Acro-osteolysis Syndromes)

Hallermann–Streiff Syndrome (see Oculomandibulo-facial Syndrome)

Holt–Oram Syndrome [142900]

Clinical features:	Congenital heart disease, abnormalities of the upper limbs, notably thumb hypoplasia, triphalangism or rarely, phocomelia.
Radiographic features:	Variable anomalies of the hands and arms, especially the thumbs.
Genetics:	AD with variable expression.
References:	Basson CT, Cowley GS, Solomons SD, Weissman B, Poznanski AK, Traill TA, Seidman CE, (1994). The clinical and genetic spectrum of the Holt–Oram syndrome (heart–hand syndrome). New Eng J Med 330:885–891

Hurst JA, Hall CM, Baraitser M (1991). The Holt–Oram syndrome. J Med Genet 28:406–410

Newbury-Ecob RA, Leanage R, Raeburn JA, Young ID (1996). Holt–Oram syndrome: a clinical genetic study. J Med Genet 33:300–307

Poznanski AK, Gall JC Jr, Stern AM (1970). Skeletal manifestations of the Holt–Oram syndrome. Radiology 94:45–53

Humerospinal Dysostosis [143095]

Clinical features:	Narrow thorax, limited elbow extension, bowing of the long bones, hyperlordosis.
Radiographic features:	Coronal cleft vertebrae, bifid distal humeral metaphyses, subluxation in the elbow joints, congenital heart disease.
Genetics:	Uncertain, very rare.
References:	Cortina H, Vidal J, Vallcanera A, Alberto C, Muro D, Dominguez F (1979). Humero-spinal dysostosis. Pediat Radiol 8:188–190
	Kozlowski KS, Celermajer JM, Tink AR (1974). Humerospinal dysostosis with congenital heart disease. Am J Dis Child 127:407
	Leroy JG, Speeckaert MT (1984) Humeroradioulnar synostosis appearing as distal humeral bifurcation in a patient with distal phocomelia of the upper limbs and radial ectrodactyly. Am J Med Genet 18:365–368

Hunter Syndrome: MPS II (see Complex Carbohydrate Metabolic Disorders)

Hurler Syndrome: MPS I-H (see Complex Carbohydrate Metabolic Disorders)

Hyperparathyroidism, Familial [239200;145807]

Clinical features:	Vary from normality to advanced biochemical and radiological manifestations.

Radiographic features: Variable bone cysts, osteoporosis, fractures, acro-osteolysis, abnormal trabecular pattern, subperiosteal erosions, tapering clavicles.

Genetics: AR; AD.

Other considerations: Hyperparathyroidism is usually non-familial but genetic neonatal [239200] and transient neonatal [145980] forms have been documented. Further heterogeneity is likely.

References: Cole DE, Janicic N, Salisbury SR, Hendy GN (1997). Neonatal severe hyperparathyroidism, secondary hyperparathyroidism, and familial hypocalciuric hypercalcemia: Am J Med Genet 71:202–210

Cronin CS, Reeve TS, Robinson B et al. (1996). Primary hyperparathyroidism in childhood and adolescence. J Paediatr Child Health 32:397–399

Kozlowski K, Czerminska-Kowalska A, Kulczycka H, Rowinska E, Pronicka E (1999). Dominantly inherited isolated hyperparathyroidism: a syndromic association? Pediatr Radiol 29:10–15

Hyperphosphatasia (see Osteoectasia with Hyperphosphatasia)

Hypochondrogenesis [120140.0007]

Clinical features: Severe short-limbed dwarfism, usually lethal in the perinatal period.

Radiographic features: Shortening of the tubular bones that have rounded ends. Platyspondyly, deficient vertebral ossification in the cervical region, short ribs, absent pubic bones and hypoplastic ilia are additional features.

Genetics: AD, new mutation (proven by molecular studies).

Other considerations: Hypochondrogenesis and achondrogenesis type II represent a continuous clinical and radiographic spectrum of the same disorder. (see 200610) Type II collagen is greatly reduced in cartilage in both conditions and mutations of the type II collagen gene (COL2A1) have been demonstrated in both disorders and in other skeletal dysplasias.

References: Maroteaux P, Stanescu V, Stanescu R (1983).
                               Hypochondrogenesis. Eur J Pediatr 141:14–22.

Hypochondroplasia [146000]

Clinical features: Resembles achondroplasia in mild degree, limb
                               shortening, normal facies, lumbar lordosis.

Radiographic features: Mild shortening of the tubular bones with minor
                               broadening of the ends of the shafts, short femor-
                               al necks, short vertebral pedicles with variable
                               caudal narrowing of the interpediculate distances.

Genetics: AD.

Other considerations: Clinical and radiographic distinction between
                               mild achondroplasia and severe hypochondropla-
                               sia can be very difficult. Mildly affected persons
                               merge with normality and frequently remain
                               undiagnosed.

References: Appan S, Laurent S, Chapman M, Hindmarsh PC,
                                   Brook CGD (1990). Growth and growth hor-
                                   mone therapy in hypochondroplasia. Acta
                                   Paediat Scand 79:796–803
                               Hall BD, Spranger J (1979). Hypochondroplasia;
                                   clinical and radiological aspects in 39 cases.
                                   Radiology 133:95–100
                               Heselson NG, Cremin BJ, Beighton P (1979). The
                                   radiographic manifestations of hypochondro-
                                   plasia. Clin Radiol 30:79–85
                               Rousseau F, Bonaventure J, Legeai-Mallet L,
                                   Schmidt H, Weissenbach J, Maroteaux P,
                                   Munnich A, Le Merrer M (1996). Clinical and
                                   genetic heterogeneity of hypochondroplasia. J
                                   Med Genet 33:749–752

Hypophosphatasia [146300; 241500]

Clinical features: Variable in severity, defective calvarial mineralis-
                               ation, later craniostenosis. Stunted stature, limb
                               bowing, skeletal fragility, low serum alkaline
                               phosphatase activity.

Radiographic features: Irregular metaphyses, bowed tubular bones.

Genetics: AD forms (heterogeneous).

Other considerations: Severe AR form is lethal in infancy [241500]. Childhood [241510] and adult varieties are milder.

References: Fallon MD, Teitelbaum SL, Weinstein RS, Goldfischer S, Brown DM, Whyte MP (1984). Hypophosphatasia: clinicopathologic comparison of the infantile, childhood, and adult forms. Medicine 63:12–24

Weinstein RS, Whyte MP (1981). Heterogeneity of adult hypophosphatasia: report of severe and mild cases. Arch Intern Med 141:727–731

Whyte MP, Murphy WA, Fallon MD (1982). Adult hypophosphatasia with chondrocalcinosis and arthropathy: variable penetrance of hypophosphatasemia in a large Oklahoma kindred. Am J Med 72:631–641

Hypophosphataemia: Vitamin D-resistant Rickets (see Rickets)

Hypopituitarism (Pituitary dwarfism) [173100; 262400; 262650]

Clinical features: Proportionate dwarfism, hypogonadism present in some forms.

Radiographic features: Delayed ossification. In putative sub-types, the sella turcica is described as large, empty or small.

Genetics: Heterogeneous: AR, AD and non-genetic forms.

Other considerations: In early reports persons with hypopituitarism were termed "midgets" or "primordial and ateliotic dwarfs". Collectively these conditions are fairly common.

References: Laron Z (1990). Hereditary dwarfism with high GH levels. Current Contents 33:24–25

Merimee TJ, Hall JG, Rimoin DL, McKusick VA (1969). A metabolic and hormonal basis for classifying ateliotic dwarfs. Lancet I:963–967

Poskitt EM, Rayner PHW (1974). Isolated growth hormone deficiency: two families with autosomal dominant inheritance. Arch Dis Child 49:55–61

Van Gelderen HH, van der Hoog CE (1981). Familial isolated growth hormone deficiency. Clin Genet 20:173–175

Hypothyroidism [218700; 274500]

Clinical features:	Mental and physical retardation due to thyroid malfunction, if untreated.
Radiographic features:	Epiphyseal stippling in infancy, delayed fusion of epiphyses, later collapse of femoral heads.
Genetics:	Heterogeneous, AR or sporadic.
Other considerations:	Common, osseous stigmata very variable. The term "cretinism" pertains to the manifestations in the untreated patient.
References:	Burke JW, Williamson BR, Hurst RW (1988). Idiopathic cerebellar calcifications: Association with hypothyroidism? Radiology 167:533–536 Eberle AJ (1993). Congenital hypothyroidism presenting as apparent spondyloepiphyseal dysplasia. Am J Med Genet 47:464–467 Nishi Y, Masuda H, Iwamori H, Urabe T, Sakoda K, Uozumi T, Usui T (1985). Primary hypothyroidism associated with pituitary enlargement, slipped capital femoral epiphysis and cystic ovaries. Eur J Pediatr 143:216–219

I-Cell Disease: MLS II (see Complex Carbohydrate Metabolic Disorders)

Idiopathic Osteolyses (see Osteolysis Syndromes)

Incontinentia Pigmenti [308300; 308310]

Clinical features:	Widespread darkly pigmented dermal lesions, inconsistent ocular defects and mental retardation, very variable skeletal changes.
Radiographic features:	Occasional structural anomalies of vertebral bodies, ribs, long bones and digits.
Genetics:	XL dominant with male lethality. Heterogeneous.

Other considerations: The skin changes overshadow the skeletal abnormalities.

References: Landy SJ, Donnai D (1993). Incontinentia pigmenti (Bloch-Sulzberger syndrome). J Med Genet 30:53–59

Parrish JE, Scheuerle AE, Lewis RA, Levy ML, Nelson DL (1996). Selection against mutant alleles in blood leukocytes is a consistent feature in incontinentia pigmenti type 2. Hum Molec Genet 5:1777–1783

Spallone A (1987). Incontinentia pigmenti (Bloch-Sulzberger syndrome): seven case reports from one family. Br J Ophthal 71:629–634

Infantile Cortical Hyperostosis (see Caffey Disease)

Jaffe–Lichtenstein Syndrome (see Fibrous Dysplasia)

Jeune Syndrome (see Asphyxiating Thoracic Dysplasia)

Juvenile Idiopathic Osteoporosis [259750]

Clinical features: Backache and progressive deformities of the spine and extremities. The disease can stabilise or remit at any stage.

Radiographic features: Generalised osteoporosis. Mild to moderate biconcave flattening of the vertebral bodies is usually evident. Fractures of the long bones are seen in more severe cases.

Genetics: Non-genetic (?).

Other considerations: This rare disorder may be difficult to distinguish from osteogenesis imperfecta and various forms of metabolic bone disease.

References: Houang MTW, Brenton DP, Renton P, Shaw DG (1978). Idiopathic juvenile osteoporosis. Skeletal Radiol 3:17–23

Smith R (1980). Idiopathic osteoporosis in the young. J Bone Joint Surg [Br] 62:417–427

Teotia M, Teotia SPS, Singh RK (1979). Idiopathic juvenile osteoporosis. Am J Dis child 133:894–900

Juvenile Paget Disease (see Osteoectasia with Hyperphosphatasia)

Kenny-Caffey Syndrome (see Tubular Stenosis)

Keutel Syndrome [245150]

Clinical features:	Pulmonary stenosis, short terminal phalanges, calcification of cartilage in the external ears, nose, larynx, trachea and ribs. Neural hearing loss.
Radiographic features:	Calcification and ossification of cartilage, as above.
Genetics:	AR, rare.
Other considerations:	May present as stippled epiphyses.
References:	Cormode EJ, Dawson M, Lowry RB (1986). Keutel syndrome: Clinical report and literature review. Am J Med Genet 24:289–294
	Khosroshahi HE, Uluoglu O, Olgunturk R, Basaklar C (1989). Keutal syndrome: a report of four cases. Europ J Pediat 149:188–191

Kleeblattschädel Syndrome (see Cloverleaf Skull)

Klinefelter Syndrome

Clinical features:	Male with hypogonadism, sometimes low intelligence, gynecomastia, "marfanoid" habitus.
Radiographic features:	Inconsistent minor changes in the length of tubular bones of digits and anomalies of ribs and spine.
Genetics:	Supernumerary X chromosome in males, i.e. XXY karyotype.
Other considerations:	The Klinefelter syndrome is common but the clinical and radiographic features may be non-specific and merge with normality. Diagnosis is established by cytogenetic studies.
References:	Ohsawa T (1971). Roentgenographic manifestations of Klinefelter's syndrome. Am J Roentgenol 112:178–184

Klippel–Feil Syndrome [148900]

Clinical features:	Short rigid neck with low hairline.
Radiographic features:	Fusion of cervical vertebrae.
Genetics:	Heterogeneous, usually non-genetic, sometimes AD.
Other considerations:	Common. Associated anomalies that may be present include cardiac defects, Sprengel shoulder and scoliosis. (see Wildervanck syndrome [3146001]).
References:	Clarke RA, Singh S, McKenzie H, Kearsley JH, Yip M-Y (1995). Familial Klippel–Feil syndrome and paracentric inversion inv(8)(q22.2q23.3). Am J Hum Genet 57:1364–1370
	Nguyen VD, Tyrrel R (1993). Klippel–Feil syndrome: patterns of bony fusion and wasp waist sign. Skeletal Radiology 22:519–523

Klippel–Trenaunay–Weber Syndrome (Angio-osteohypertrophy) [149000]

Clinical features:	Asymmetrical overgrowth of one or more limbs, sometimes with involvement of the trunk and head. Superficial and deep angiomatous malformations are syndromic components.
Radiographic features:	Bony overgrowth and malformation in the affected parts. No vascular lesions in bone.
Genetics:	Probably non-genetic. Distinction from Proteus syndrome [176920] may be difficult.
References:	Phillips GN, Gordon DH, Martin EC, Jack OH, Casarella W (1978). The Klippel-Trenaunay syndrome: clinical and radiological aspects. Radiology 128:429–434
	Samuel M, Spitz L (1995). Klippel-Trenaunay syndrome: clinical features, complications and management in children. Br J Surg 82:757–761
	Viljoen DL (1988). Klippel–Trenaunay–Weber syndrome (angio-osteohypertrophy syndrome). J Med Genet 25:250–252

Kniest Dysplasia (Metatropic Dysplasia Type II) [156550]

Clinical features:	Short trunk, short limb dwarfism, severe kyphoscoliosis, flat face, deafness, myopia, retinal detachment, stiff knobbly joints.
Radiographic features:	Platyspondyly, delayed ossification of femoral capital epiphyses, broad metaphyses, bulky epiphyses, metacarpal pseudo-epiphyses.
Genetics:	AD.
Other considerations:	Kniest dysplasia must be differentiated from metatropic dysplasia type I, an AR disorder [250600]. Burton dysplasia [245160] resembles Kniest dysplasia, but can be differentiated on a basis of radiological features and the AR mode of inheritance.
References:	Gilbert-Barnes E, Langer LO Jr, Opitz JM, Laxova R, Sotelo-Arila C (1996). Kniest dysplasia: radiologic, histopathological, and scanning electronmicroscopic findings. Am J Med Genet 63:34–45
	Lo IFM, Roebuck DJ, Lam STS, Kozlowski K (1998). Burton skeletal dysplasia: the second case report. Am J Med Genet 79:168–171
	Spranger J, Winterpacht A, Zabel B (1997). Kniest dysplasia: Dr W Kniest, his patient, the molecular defect. Am J Med Genet 69:79–84
	Wilkin DJ, Artz AS, South S, Lachman RS, Rimoin DL, Wilcox WR, McKusick VA, Stratakis CA, Francomano CA, Cohn DH (1999). Small deletions in the Type II collagen triple helix produce Kniest dysplasia. Am J Med Genet 85:105–112

Kosenow-Sinios Syndrome (see Scapuloiliac Dysplasia)

Kyphomelic Dysplasia [211350]

Clinical features:	Congenital bowing of the limb bones, predominantly the femora. Dimples may be present in the mid-thighs, over the apices of the angulations.
Radiographic features:	The femora are short, broad and bent with mild metaphyseal irregularity.

Genetics: AR.

Other considerations: Kyphomelic dysplasia must be distinguished from campomelic dysplasia. In the latter condition the tubular bones are thin but not shortened and significant involvement of the tibiae is present. The Stuve-Wiedemann syndrome [601559] is a similar AR disorder in which digital contractures and metaphyseal widening are additional features.

References:

Cormier-Daire V, Munnich A, Lyonnet S, Rustin P, Delezoide AL, Maroteaux P, Le Merrer M (1998). Presentation of six cases of Stüve-Wiedemann syndrome. Pediatr Radiol 28:776–780

Kozlowski K, Tenconi R (1996). Stuve-Wiedemann dysplasia in a 3.5 year old boy. Am J Med Genet 63:17–19

Turnpenny PD, Dakwar RA, Boulos FN (1990). Kyphomelic dysplasia: the first 10 cases. J Med Genet 27:269–272

Viljoen D, Beighton P (1988). Kyphomelic dysplasia: further delineation of the phenotype. Dysmorph Clin Genet 1:136–141

Wiedemann H-R, Stuve A (1996). Stuve-Wiedemann syndrome: update and historical footnote. Am J Med Genet 63:12–16

La Chappelle Dysplasia (see Atelosteogenesis Type II)

Langer Type of Mesomelic Dysplasia (see Mesomelic Dysplasia)

Langer–Saldino Dysplasia (see Achondrogenesis Type II)

Larsen Syndrome [150250; 245600]

Clinical features: Stunted stature, multiple joint dislocations, especially knees, hips and radial heads, dish face, spatulate terminal phalanges.

Radiographic features: Dislocations, subluxations and spinal malalignment, inconsistent vertebral anomalies in the thoracic region, double ossification centre in the calcaneum, supernumerary carpal bones.

Genetics: AD – mild. AR – severe. Heterogeneous.

Other considerations: Probably under-diagnosed. An AR variant form is present in a high frequency on the Island of Reunion. Another severe AR form is lethal in the newborn.

References: Bonaventure J, Lasselin C, Mellier J, Cohen-Solal L, Maroteaux P (1992). Linkage studies of four fibrillar collagen genes in three pedigrees with Larsen-like syndrome. J Med Genet 29:465–470

Johnston CE II, Birch JG, Daniels JL (1996). Cervical kyphosis in patients who have Larsen syndrome. J Bone Joint Surg 78A:538–545

Kozlowski K, Robertson F, Middleton R (1974). Radiographic findings in Larsen's syndrome. Australas Radiol 18:336–344

Laville JM, Lakermance P, Limouzy F (1994). Larsen's syndrome: review of the literature and analysis of 38 cases. J Ped Orthop 14:63–73

Lenz–Majewski Dysplasia [151050]

Clinical features: Dwarfism, patent fontanelles, hypertelorism, choanal stenosis, dental abnormalities, lax joints, mental retardation. Progeroid appearance.

Radiographic features: Sclerosis of skull, facial bones and vertebrae; sclerosis of cortices of tubular bones; broad clavicles and ribs; short middle phalanges.

Genetics: Sporadic. New dominant mutation?

Other considerations: Very rare.

References: Chrzanowska KH, Fryns JP, Krajewska-Walasek M, Van den Berghe H, Wisniewski L (1989). Skeletal dysplasia syndrome with progeroid appearance, characteristic facial and limb anomalies, multiple synostoses, and distinct skeletal changes: a variant example of the Lenz–Majewski syndrome. Am J Med Genet 32:470–474

Gorlin RJ, Whitley CB (1983). Lenz–Majewski syndrome. Radiology 149:129–131

Leroy I-Cell Disease: MLS II (see Complex Carbohydrate
Metabolic Disorders)

Lobster-Claw Malformation (see Ectrodactyly)

Maffucci Syndrome (see Enchondromatosis with
Haemangiomata)

Majewski Syndrome (see Short Rib Syndrome Type II)

Mandibulofacial Dysostosis (see Treacher Collins Syndrome)

Mannosidosis (see Complex Carbohydrate Metabolic
Disorders)

Marfan Syndrome [154700]

Clinical features:	Tall stature with excessive limb length and arachnodactyly, variable dislocation of ocular lenses, high palate, aortic and mitral valve incompetence, sternal asymmetry and spinal malalignment, high incidence of dissection of the aorta.
Radiographic features:	Excessive length of tubular bones of extremities in relation to their width (the numerical value of the metacarpal index reflects this feature).
Genetics:	AD with variable expression.
Other considerations:	The Marfan syndrome is comparatively common but patients with incomplete manifestations abound and firm diagnosis may be difficult. Congenital contractural arachnodactyly (Beals syndrome [121050]) has the additional features of digital contractures and crumpled ears. Shprintzen-Goldberg syndrome [182212] is a similar progressive disorder.
References:	Gray JR, Davies SJ (1996). Marfan syndrome. J Med Genet 33:403–408
	Robinson PN, Godfrey M (2000). The molecular genetics of Marfan syndrome and related microfibrillopathies. J Med Genet 37:9–25

Seemanova E, Kozlowski K (1997). Shprintzen-Goldberg syndrome. Radiol Med 94:673–675

Tallroth K, Malmivaara A, Laitinen M-L, Savolainen A, Harilainen A (1995). Lumbar spine in Marfan syndrome. Skeletal Radiol 24:337–340

Viljoen D, Beighton P (1990). Marfan syndrome: a diagnostic dilemma. Clin Genet 37:417–422

Maroteaux–Lamy Syndrome: MPS IV (see Complex Carbohydrate Metabolic Disorders)

Marshall Syndrome [154780]

Clinical features: Accelerated linear growth with failure to thrive, retarded motor and mental development, peculiar facies, early death from pneumonia. The hair and teeth are sometimes dysplastic.

Radiographic features: Advanced bone age.

Genetics: Unknown.

Other considerations: Rare. Identity with the Wagner [143200] and Stickler [108300] syndromes is possible. The presence of ectodermal dysplasia in Marshall syndrome is a distinguishing feature.

References:
Ayme S, Preus M (1984). The Marshall and Stickler syndromes: objective rejection of lumping. J Med Genet 21:34–38

Shanske AL, Bogdanow A, Shprintzen RJ, Marion RW (1997). The Marshall syndrome: report of a new family and review of the literature. Am J Med Genet 70:52–57

Stratton RF, Lee B, Ramirez F (1991). Marshall syndrome. Am J Med Genet 41:35–38

Maxillonasal Dysplasia (see Binder syndrome)

McCune–Albright Syndrome (see Fibrous Dysplasia)

Melnick–Needles Syndrome (see Osteodysplasty)

Melorheostosis [155950]

Clinical features: Asymptomatic or localised pain with sclerotic dermal changes and joint contractures.

Radiographic features: Unilateral, irregular, linear areas of increased density, which appear to be "flowing", down the long axes of the tubular bones.

Genetics: Non-genetic.

Other considerations: Post-zygotic mutation may be the pathogenetical mechanism.

References: Campbell CJ, Papademetriou T, Bonfiglio M (1968). Melorheostosis. A report of the clinical, roentgenographic and pathological findings in fourteen cases. J Bone Joint Surg [Am] 50:1281–1304

Nevin NC, Thomas PS, Davis RI, Cowie GH (1999). Melorheostosis in a family with auto-somal dominant osteopoikilosis. Am J Med Genet 82:409–414

Rhys R, Davies AM, Mangham DC, Grimer RJ (1998). Sclerotome distribution of melorheos-tosis and multicentric fibromatosis. Skeletal Radiol 27:633–636

Yu JS, Resnick D, Vaughan LM, Haghighi P, Hughes T (1995). Melorheostosis with an ossified soft tissue mass: MR features. Skeletal Radiol 24:367–370

Menkes Kinky Hair Syndrome [309400]

Clinical features: Deficient growth, progressive central nervous degeneration, sparse light hair, death in infancy.

Radiographic features: Osteoporosis, rickets-like changes with spur formation, metaphyseal fractures, multiple worm-ian bones.

Genetics: XL.

Other considerations: Skeletal changes have been confused with those of the battered baby syndrome and infantile nutri-tional copper deficiency.

References: Danks DM, Stevens BJ, Campbell PE (1972). Menkes kinky hair syndrome. Lancet I:1100–1106

Kozlowski K, McCrossin R (1980). Early osseous abnormalities in Menkes kinky hair syndrome. Pediatr Radiol 8:191–194

Proud VK, Mussell HG, Kaler SG, Young DW, Percy AK (1996). Distinctive Menkes disease variant with occipital horns: delineation of natural history and clinical phenotype. Am J Med Genet 65:44–51

Mesomelic Dysplasia

The mesomelic dysplasias are rare but very heterogeneous. The best known forms are summarised below:

General References: Kaitila II, Leisti JT, Rimoin DL (1976). Mesomelic skeletal dysplasias. Clin Orthop Rel Res 114:94–99

Maroteaux P, Spranger J (1977). Essai de classification des chondrodysplasies à prédominance mésomélique. Arch Fr Pediatr 34:945–949

Silverman FN (1973). Mesomelic dwarfism. In: Prog Pediatr Radiol, vol 4, Intrinsic diseases of bones. Karger, Basel, pp 546–562

1. Acromesomelic Dysplasia [201250]

Clinical features: Dwarfism with shortening of the middle segments of the limbs and digits.

Radiographic features: Short middle and distal segments of the extremities, Variable platyspondyly.

Genetics: AR. Heterogeneous.

Other considerations: It is uncertain whether the "Maroteaux" and "Campailla–Martinelli" forms are the same, or distinct. Other conditions with significant acromesomelia include Weill–Marchesani dysplasia [277600], Cranioectodermal dysplasia [218330] and Hunter-Thompson dysplasia [201250].

References: Beighton P (1974). Autosomal recessive inheritance in the mesomelic dwarfism of Campailla and Martinelli. Clin Genet 5:363–367

Langer LO, Beals RK, Solomon IL, Bard PA, Bard LA, Rissman EM, Rogers JG, Dorst JP, Hall JG, Sparkes RS, Franken EA (1977). Acromesomelic dwarfism: manifestations in childhood. Am J Med Genet 1:87–100

Langer LO, Cervanka J, Camargo M (1989). A severe autosomal recessive acromesomelic dysplasia, the Hunter-Thompson type, and comparison with the Grebe type. Hum Genet 81:323–328

2. Nievergelt Type [163400]

Clinical features: Dwarfism with forearm and leg deformities.

Radiographic features: Rhomboid-shaped forearm and leg bones, multiple radio-ulnar, tarsal and carpal synostoses.

Genetics: AD, rare.

References: Hess OM, Goebel NH, Streuli R (1978). Familiaerer mesomeler Kleinwuchs (Nievergelt-Syndrom). Schweiz Med Wschr 108:1202–1206

Young LW, Wood BP (1975). Nievergelt syndrome. Birth Defects: Original Articles Series 11(5):81–85

3. Robinow Type [180700]

Clinical features: Dwarfism with forearm shortening, craniofacial dysmorphism, abnormal external genitalia.

Radiographic features: Shortening of the medial segments of the extremities, malsegmentation of the spine.

Genetics: AD; AR form?

References: Aksit S, Aydinlioglu H, Dizdarer G, Caglayan S, Bektaslar D, Cin A (1997). Is the frequency of Robinow syndrome relatively high in Turkey? Four more case reports. Clin Genet 52:226–230

Butler MG, Wadlington WB (1987). Robinow syndrome: report of two cases and review of literature. Clin Genet 31:77–85

Kantaputra PN, Gorlin RJ, Ukarapol N, Unachak K, Sudasna J (1999). Robinow (fetal face) syndrome: report of a boy with dominant type and an infant with recessive type. Am J Med Genet 84:1–7

4. Langer Type [249700]

Clinical features: Mesomelic dwarfism, mandibular hypoplasia.

Radiographic features:	Shortening, hypoplasia and deformity of the medial segments of the extremities.
Genetics:	AR.
Other considerations:	This rare disorder represents the homozygous state of the single gene autosomal dominant disorder, dyschondrosteosis [127300]. In this way, both parents and all offspring of a person with Langer mesomelic dwarfism necessarily have dyschondrosteosis.
References:	Espiritu C, Chen H, Wooley PV (1975). Mesomelic dwarfism as the homozygous expression of dyschondrosteosis. Am J Dis Child 129:375–380
	Goldblatt J, Wallis C, Viljoen D, Beighton P (1987). Heterozygous manifestations of Langer mesomelic dysplasia. Clin Genet 31:19–24
	Kunze J, Klemm T (1980). Mesomelic dysplasia, type Langer – a homozygous state for dyschondrosteosis. Eur J Pediatr 134:269–272

5. Rheinhardt–Pfeiffer Type

Clinical features:	Short stature, forearm bowing with shortening of the fibulae.
Radiographic features:	Distal ulnar and proximal fibular hypoplasia.
Genetics:	AD.
Other considerations:	Syndromic identity is uncertain.
References:	Rheinhardt K, Pfeiffer RA (1967). Ulno-fibulare dysplasie. Eine autosomal-dominant vererbte Mikromesomelie ähnlich dem Nievergelts Syndrom. Fortsch Roentgenstr 107:379–384

6. Hypoplastic Tibia and Radius Type [156230]

Clinical features:	Stunted stature, secondary to shortening of the legs, polydactyly, absent thumbs.
Radiographic features:	Aplasia of tibia and patella, relatively normal fibula, variable hypoplasia of metatarsals and phalanges.
Genetics:	AD.

References: Leroy J (1975). Dominant mesomelic dwarfism of
                          the hypoplastic tibia, radius type. Clin Genet
                          7:280–285

7. Werner Type

Clinical features: Stunted stature, gross tibial hypoplasia, absence
                          of the thumb.

Radiographic features: as above.

Genetics: AD.

Other Considerations: Werner syndrome is a different entity [277700].

References: Pashayan H, Fraser FC, McIntyre JM, Dunbar JS
                          (1971). Bilateral aplasia of the tibia, polydactyly
                          and absent thumbs in father and daughter. J
                          Bone Jt Surg 53B:495–499

8. Mesomelic Dysplasia with Synostoses

Clinical features: Stunted stature, characteristic facies, short digits.

Radiographic features: Severe metaphyseal change in the limbs. Synos-
                          toses in the extremities.

Genetics: AD.

Other considerations: Very rare.

References: Pfeiffer RA, Hirschfelder H, Rott HD (1995).
                          Specific acromesomelia with facial and renal
                          anomalies: a new syndrome. Clin Dysmorph
                          4:38–43
                          Verloes A, David A (1995). Dominant mesomelic
                          shortness of stature with acral synostoses,
                          umbilical anomalies, and soft palate agenesis.
                          Am J Med Genet 55:205–212

9. Mesomelic Dysplasia – Other Forms

Other uncommon mesomelic dysplasia are referenced below:

                          Kerner B, Rimoin DL, Lachman RS (1998).
                          Mesomelic shortening of the upper extremities
                          with spur formation and cutaneous dimpling.
                          Pediatr Radiol 28:794–797
                          Reardon W, Hall CM, Slaney S, Huson SM,
                          Connell J, Al-Hilaly N, Fixsen J, Baraitser M,
                          Winter RM (1993). Mesomelic limb shortness:

a previously unreported autosomal recessive type. Am J Med Genet 47:788–792

Metachondromatosis [156250]

Clinical features: Juxta-articular swellings predominantly in the hands and feet.

Radiographic features: Exostoses and enchondromata around the digital joints.

Genetics: AD.

Other considerations: This uncommon disorder may be misdiagnosed as diaphyseal aclasis or multiple cartilaginous exostoses.

References: Bassett GS, Cowell HR (1985). Metachondromatosis: report of four cases. J Bone Joint Surg 67A:811–814

Kozlowski K, Scougall JS (1975). Metachondromatosis: report of a case in a six year old boy. Aust Paediatr J 11(1):42–47

Metaphyseal Chondrodysplasia with Pancreatic Insufficiency and Bone Marrow Dysfunction (Shwachman Syndrome) [260400]

Clinical features: Short stature, ectodermal dysplasia, chronic bacterial infections, lymphopenia, agammaglobulinaemia, thymic hypoplasia.

Radiographic features: Shortening of the tubular bones with widening of the metaphyses, narrow sacro-iliac notches, low acetabular angles.

Genetics: AR.

Other considerations: Haematological and metabolic problems predominate in this rare disorder.

References: Aggett PJ, Cavanagh NP, Matthew DJ, Pincott SR, Sutcliffe J, Harries JT (1980). Shwachman's syndrome: A review of 21 cases. Arch Dis Child 55:331–347

Mack DR, Forstner GG, Wilschanski M, Freedman MH, Durie PR (1996). Shwachman syndrome:

exocrine pancreatic dysfunction and variable phenotypic expression. Gastroenterology 111:1593–1602

McLennan TW, Steinbach HL (1974). Shwachman's syndrome: a broad spectrum of bony abnormalities. Radiology 112:167–173

Metaphyseal Chondrodysplasia, Jansen Type [156400]

Clinical features: Short-limb dwarfism with prominent joints and restricted mobility, large skull.

Radiographic features: Severe progressive metaphyseal dysplasia, normal spine and epiphyses, hyperostosis of the base of the skull.

Genetics: AD.

Other considerations: Rare but well known.

References: Holthusen W, Holt JF, Stoeckenius M (1975). The skull in metaphyseal chondrodysplasia type Jansen. Pediatr Radiol 3:137–144

Charrow J, Poznanski AK (1984). The Jansen type of metaphyseal chondrodysplasia: confirmation of dominant inheritance and review of radiographic manifestations in the newborn and adult. Am J Med Genet 18:321–327

Metaphyseal Chondrodysplasia, McKusick Type (Cartilage-Hair Hypoplasia) [250250]

Clinical features: Short-limbed dwarfism, fine sparse hair, stubby digits. Megacolon and immunological incompetence are sometimes present.

Radiographic features: Shortening of the tubular bones, metaphyseal "cupping" maximal in the hips and knees, normal skull. Delayed skeletal age. Distal prolongation of the fibula. Ribs flared anteriorly.

Genetics: AR.

Other considerations: This disorder is most prevalent in the Amish religious isolate of Pennsylvania and in Finland.

References: Makitie O, Marttinen E, Kaitila I (1992). Skeletal growth in cartilage-hair hypoplasia – a radiological study of 82 patients. Pediat Radiol 22:434–439

Sulisalo T, Mäkitie O, Sistonen P, Ridanpää M, El-Rifai W, Ruuskanen O, de la Chapelle A, Kaitila I (1996). Uniparental disomy in cartilage-hair hypoplasia. Eur J Hum Genet 5:35–42

Van der Burgt I, Haraldsson A, Oosterwijk JC, van Essen AJ, Weemaes C, Hamel B (1991). Cartilage hair hypoplasia, metaphyseal chondrodysplasia type McKusick: description of seven patients and review of the literature. Am J Med Genet 41:371–380

Metaphyseal Chondrodysplasia, Schmid Type [156500]

Clinical features: Small stature, bowed legs.

Radiographic features: Shortened tubular bones, moderate metaphyseal dysplasia, most severe in the knees and hips, coxa vara.

Genetics: AD.

Other considerations: This condition is by far the most common of the metaphyseal dysplasias.

References: Lachman RS, Rimoin DL, Spranger J (1988). Metaphyseal chondrodysplasia, Schmid type: clinical and radiographic delineation with a review of the literature. Pediat Radiol 18:93–102

Wallis GA, Rash B, Sykes B, Bonaventure J, Maroteaux P, Zabel B, Wynne-Davies R, Grant ME, Boot-Handford RP (1996). Mutations within the gene encoding the alpha-1(X) chain type X collagen (COL1A1) cause metaphyseal chondrodysplasia type Schmid but not several other forms of chondrodysplasia. J Med Genet 33:450–457

Metaphyseal Chondrodysplasia, Other Forms

Clinical features: Involvement of the metaphyses is the main feature of several rare bone dysplasias, including the Spahr type of metaphyseal dysplasia [250400], various forms of acroscyphodysplasia [250215] and metaphyseal anadysplasia [309645].

References:

Joquier S, Bellini F, Mackensie DA (1981). Metaphyseal chondrodysplasia with ectodermal dysplasia. Skeletal Radiol 7:107–112

Le Merrer M, Maroteaux P (1998). Metaphyseal anadysplasia type II: a new regressive metaphyseal dysplasia. Pediatr Radiol 28:771–775

Nishimura G, Kozlowski K (1993). Osteosclerotic metaphyseal dysplasia. Pediatr Radiol 23:450–452

Metaphyseal Dysplasia (Pyle Dysplasia) [265900]

Clinical features:

Asymptomatic or may involve minor limb deformities, notably genu valgus. Articular pains and fractures are occasional features.

Radiographic features:

Gross metaphyseal flaring of the long bones, maximal at the knees. Some expansion of the flat bones and the ribs, moderate sclerosis of the skull.

Genetics:

AR.

Other considerations:

The innocuous clinical features contrast with the striking radiological changes. Semantic confusion exists with the cranio-metaphyseal dysplasias, which are separate entities.

References:

Beighton P (1987). Pyle disease (metaphyseal dysplasia). J Med Genet 24:321–324

Heselson NG, Raad MS, Hamersma H, Cremin B, Beighton P (1979). The radiological manifestations of metaphyseal dysplasia (Pyle disease). Br J Radiol 52:431–437

Metatropic Dysplasia Type I [250600]

Clinical features:

Initially short extremities and long trunk, changing into short-trunk dwarfism later in life, prominent joints with restricted movements, tail-like sacral appendage.

Radiographic features: Characteristic platyspondyly, tubular bones have broad metaphyses and dysplastic epiphyses.

Genetics: AR; heterogeneous.

Other considerations: Uncommon but well delineated. (see Metatropic dysplasia type II, Kniest dysplasia [156550]).

References:

Beck M, Roubicek M, Rogers JG, Naumoff P, Spranger J (1983). Heterogeneity of metatropic dysplasia. Eur J Pediat 140:231–237

Boden SD, Kaplan FS, Fallon MD, Ruddy R, Belik J, Anday E, Zackai E, Ellis J (1987). Metatropic dwarfism: uncoupling of endochondral and perichondral growth. J Bone Joint Surg 69A:174–184

Kozlowski K, Morris L, Reinwein H, Sprague P, Tamaela LA (1976). Metatropic dwarfism and its variants. Australas Radiol 20:367–385

Metatropic Dysplasia Type II (see Kniest Syndrome)

Meyer Dysplasia (see Perthes Disease)

Micrognathic Dwarfism (see Weissenbacher and Zweymuller Syndrome)

Mohr Syndrome (see Oro-facial-digital Syndrome)

Morquio Syndrome: MPS IV (see Complex Carbohydrate Metabolic Disorders)

Mucolipidoses (MLS) (see Complex Carbohydrate Metabolic Disorders)

Mucopolysaccharidoses (see Complex Carbohydrate Metabolic Disorders)

Mucosulfatidosis (see Complex Carbohydrate Metabolic Disorders)

Multiple Cartilaginous Exostoses (Diaphyseal Aclasis) [133700; 133701; 600209]

Clinical features: Multiple protuberances at the ends of tubular bones, ribs, scapulae and ilia. Limb deformity, particularly of the forearms. Stunted stature.

Radiographic features: Multiple exostoses with secondary deformity of the tubular and flat bones. The cranium is not involved.

Genetics: AD, heterogeneous.

Other considerations: Common.

References: Epstein DA, Levin EJ (1978). Bone scintigraphy in hereditary multiple exostoses. Am J Roentgenol 130:331–336

Legeai-Mallet L, Munnich A, Maroteaux P, Le Merrer M (1997). Incomplete penetrance and expressivity skewing in hereditary multiple exostoses. Clin Genet 52:12–16

Shapiro F, Simon S, Glimcher MJ (1979). Hereditary multiple exostoses: anthropometric, roentgenographic and clinical aspects. J Bone Joint Surg 61A:815–824

Wicklund CL, Pauli RM, Johnston D, Hecht JT (1995). Natural history study of hereditary multiple exostoses. Am J Med Genet 55:43–46

Multiple Epiphyseal Dysplasia (MED) [132400; 600204]

Clinical features: Mild shortening of stature, stubby terminal phalanges in some forms.

Radiographic features: Irregular, small epiphyses, variable mild platyspondyly, premature degenerative arthropathy, especially in the hips.

Genetics: Heterogeneous. AD forms – common. AR forms – rare.

Other considerations: MED, which is loosely categorised into mild Ribbing and severe Fairbank types, enters into the differential diagnosis of any child presenting with atypical Perthes disease.

References: Ballo R, Briggs MD, Cohn DH, Knowlton RG, Beighton PH, Ramesar RS (1997). Multiple epiphyseal dysplasia, Ribbing type: a novel point mutation in the COMP gene in a South African family. Am J Med Genet 68:396–400

Kozlowski K, Lipska K (1967). Hereditary dysplasia epiphysealis multiplex. Clin Radiol 18:330–336

Oehlmann R. Summerville GP, Yeh G, Weaver EJ, Jimenez SA, Knowlton RG (1994). Genetic linkage mapping of multiple epiphyseal dysplasia to the pericentromeric region of chromosome 19. Am J Hum Genet 54:3–10

Superti-Furga A, Neumann L, Riebel T, Eich G, Steinmann B, Spranger J, Kunze J (1999). Recessively inherited multiple epiphyseal dysplasia with normal stature, clubfoot, and double layered patella caused by a DTDST mutation. J Med Genet 36:621–624

Multiple Pterygium Syndrome [265000]

Clinical features: Small stature, peculiar facies, micrognathia, pterygia (webbing) of neck, axillae, elbows and knees.

Radiographic features: Vertebral and rib abnormalities, scoliosis, hip dislocation.

Genetics: AR; heterogeneous.

Other considerations: The pterygia, which may cause considerable disability, overshadow the skeletal abnormalities. There is some nosological confusion with other rare syndromes in which pterygia are a component.

References: Ramer JC, Ladda RL, Demuth WW(1988). Multiple pterygium syndrome: an overview. Am J Dis Child 142:794–798

Spranger S, Spranger M, Meinck H-M, Tariverdian G (1995). Two sisters with Escobar syndrome. Am J Med Genet 57:425–428

Thompson EM, Donnai D, Baraitser M, Hall CM, Pembrey ME, Fixsen J (1987). Multiple pterygium syndrome: evolution of the phenotype. J Med Genet 24:733–749

Multiple Synostoses Syndrome [186400; 186500]

Clinical features: Stiff joints, usually fingers and elbows, hypoplasia of distal phalanges, conductive deafness in some families.

Radiographic features: Multiple fusions, predominantly phalangeal, carpal, tarsal and radiohumeral.

Genetics: AD with variable expression.

Other considerations: This uncommon syndrome must be distinguished from other disorders in which symphalangism occurs.

References: Da Silva EO, Filho SM, de Albuquerque SC (1984). Multiple synostosis syndrome: study of a large Brazilian kindred. Am J Med Genet 18:237–247
                         Hurvitz SA, Goodman RM, Hertz M, Katznelson MB-M, Sack Y (1985). The facio-audio-symphalangism syndrome: report of a case and review of the literature. Clin Genet 28:61–68

MURCS Association [223340]

Clinical features: Muellerian duct (genitourinary), renal and cervico-thoracic vertebral abnormalities, small stature.

Radiographic features: Fusions and structural abnormalities of cervical and thoracic vertebrae.

Genetics: Unknown.

Other considerations: The MURCS (muellerian duct, renal and cervical defects) and the VATER or VACTERL associations [192350] (vertebral abnormalities, anal atresia, tracheo-esophageal fistula with radial and renal dysplasia) are similar, but skeletal involvement in the latter is usually in the lower spine, while limb defects may also be present.

References: Lin HJ, Cornford ME, Hu B, Rutgers JKL, Beall MH, Lachman RS (1996). Occipital encephalocele and MURCS association: case report and review of central nervous system anomalies in MURCS patients. Am J Med Genet 61:59–62

Martínez-Frías M, Frías JL (1999). VACTERL as primary, polytopic developmental field defects. Am J Med Genet 83:13–16

Nezarati MM, McLeod DR (1999). VACTERL manifestations in two generations of a family. Am J Med Genet 82:40–42

Weaver DD, Mapstone CL, Yu P (1986). The VATER association: analysis of 46 patients. Am J Dis Child 140:225–229

Myhre Syndrome [139210]

Clinical features:	Short stature, low birthweight, blepharophimosis, maxillary hypoplasia, prognathism, muscle hypertrophy, stiff joints, mental retardation, deafness.
Radiographic features:	Thick calvarium, broad ribs, hypoplastic iliac wings, platyspondyly, large vertebrae, short tubular bones.
Genetics:	AD?
Other considerations:	Very rare.
References:	Garcia-Cruz D, Figuera LE, Feria-Velazco A, Sanchez-Corona J, Garcia-Cruz MO, Ramirez-Duenas RM, Hernandez-Cordova A, Ruiz MX, Bitar-Alatorre WE, Ramirez-Duenas ML, Cantu JM (1993). The Myhre syndrome: report of two cases. Clin Genet 44:203–207
	Myhre SA, Ruvalcaba R, Graham CB (1981). A new growth deficiency syndrome. Clin Genet 20:1–5

Myofibromatosis (see Fibrous Dysplasia, Congenital Generalised Form)

Myotonic Chondrodysplasia (Schwartz Syndrome) [255800; 258480]

Clinical features:	Short stature, myotonia with immobile facies, blepharophimosis, limb malalignment, kyphosis.
Radiographic features:	Dysplastic changes in all components of the spine, limbs and extremities.

Genetics:	AR; heterogeneous.
Other considerations:	About 30 patients have been reported. There is some terminological confusion but the eponym "Schwartz syndrome" has gained wide acceptance. Subdivision into mild and severe forms has been proposed.
References:	Giedion A, Boltshauser E, Briner J, Eich G, Exner G, Fendel H, Kaufmann L, Steinmann B, Spranger J, Superti-Furga A (1997). Heterogeneity in Schwartz–Jampel chondrodystrophic myotonia. Europ J Pediat 156:214–223
	Nicole S, White PS, Topaloglu H, Beighton P, Salih M, Hentati F, Fontaine B (1999). The human CDC42 gene: genomic organization, evidence for the existence of a putative pseudogene and exclusion as a SJS1 candidate gene. Hum Genet 105(1–2):98–103
	Viljoen D, Beighton P (1992). Schwartz–Jampel syndrome (chondrodystrophic myotonia). J Med Genet 29:58–62

Naevoid Basal Cell Carcinoma (see Basal Cell Naevus Carcinoma Syndrome)

Nail-Patella Syndrome (Osteo-onychodysplasia) [161200]

Clinical features:	Nail dysplasia, lack of full extension of elbows, eventual renal failure.
Radiographic features:	Hypoplastic or absent patellae, iliac horns. Mild but widespread dysplastic changes may be present, maximal in the elbows and feet.
Genetics:	AD.
Other considerations:	The syndrome is fairly common and the iliac horns are pathognomonic.
References:	Fiedler BS, De Smet AA, Kling TF Jr, Fisher DR (1987). Foot deformity in hereditary onycho-osteodysplasia. J Can Assoc Radiol 38:305–308
	Rizzo R, Pavone L, Micali G, Hall JG (1993). Familial bilateral antecubital pterygia with severe renal involvement in nail-patella syndrome. Clin Genet 44:1–7

Williams HJ, Hoyer JR (1973). Radiographic diagnosis of osteo-onychodysostosis in infancy. Radiology 109:151–154

Neurofibromatosis (von Recklinghausen Disease) [162200]

Clinical features: "Café-au-lait" macules, pedunculated and sessile cutaneous tumours, sometimes limb or digital asymmetry, kyphoscoliosis and pseudoarthrosis of the tibia.

Radiographic features: Inconsistent skeletal abnormalities – tibial pseudoarthrosis, progressive kyphoscoliosis with vertebral angulation, gigantism of the extremities with bone hypertrophy.

Genetics: AD with variable expression.

Other considerations: Very common and clinically important. Radiographic changes are not pathognomonic and in mild sporadic cases, diagnosis may be difficult. Neurofibromatosis type 2 is a different disorder, in which acoustic neuromata are a major feature.

References: Dugoff L, Sujansky E (1996). Neurofibromatosis type 1 and pregnancy. Am J Med Genet 66:7–10
Holt JF (1978). Neurofibromatosis in children. Am J Roentgen 130:615–639
McGaughran JM, Harris DI, Donnai D, Teare D, McLeod R, Westerbeek R, Kingston H, Super M, Evans DGR (1999). A clinical study of type 1 neurofibromatosis in northwest England. J Med Genet 36:197–203
Riccardi VM, Eichner JE (1986). Neurofibromatosis: Phenotype, Natural History and Pathogenesis. Baltimore: Johns Hopkins Univ Press

Nievergelt Type of Mesomelic Dysplasia (see Mesomelic Dysplasia)

Noonan-like Multiple Giant Cell Lesion Syndrome [163955]

Clinical features: Short stature, hypertelorism, prominent ears, short webbed neck, cubitus valgus, pulmonic stenosis, multiple lentigines and giant cell lesions of bone and soft tissues.

Radiographic features: Multiple radiolucent areas in mandibles and other bones.

Genetics: AD?

Other considerations: Rare, differs from the classical Noonan syndrome, which is much more common, by virtue of the osseous involvement.

References: Cohen MM, Gorlin RJ (1991). Noonan-like/ multiple giant cell lesion syndrome. Am J Med Genet 40:159–166

Ochronosis (see Alkaptonuria)

Oculoauriculo-vertebral Dysplasia (see Goldenhar Syndrome)

Oculodento-osseous Dysplasia (Oculodento-digital Dysplasia) [257850; 164200]

Clinical features: Microphthalmia, dental enamel hypoplasia, hypotrichosis, flexion and syndactyly of the 4th and 5th fingers.

Radiographic features: Hypoplasia of middle phalanx of the 5th finger. Some patients have variable skeletal sclerosis that may be severe in the skull, with gross clavicular expansion. Intracranial calcification is a feature of the severe AR form.

Genetics: Mild AD form with very variable expression. Severe AR form with expression in the heterozygote (rare).

Other considerations: This condition bears some resemblance to the Hallerman-Streiff syndrome [234100].

References: Barnard A, Hamersma H, De Villiers JC, Beighton P (1981). Intracranial calcification in oculodento-osseous dysplasia. S Afr Med J 59:758–762

Beighton P, Hamersma H, Raad M (1979). Oculodento-osseous dysplasia: heterogeneity or variable expression? Clin Genet 16:169–117

Norton KK, Carey JC, Gutmann DH (1995). Oculodentodigital dysplasia with cerebral white matter abnormalities in a two-generation family. Am J Med Genet 57:458–461

Patton MA, Laurence KM (1985). Three new cases of oculodentodigital (ODD) syndrome: development of the facial phenotype. J Med Genet 22:386–389

Oculomandibulo-facial Syndrome (Hallermann–Streiff Syndrome) [234100]

Clinical features: Shortened stature, microphthalmia, cataracts, micrognathia, frontal bossing and a narrow hooked nose.

Radiographic features: Thin bones, particularly the ribs, hypoplasia of the mandible, delayed ossification of the skull.

Genetics: AD.

Other considerations: About 100 patients have been recognised. The majority are sporadic and may represent new gene mutations. A severe form with perinatal lethality has been proposed.

References: Christian CL, Lachman RS, Aylsworth AS, Fujimoto A, Gorlin RJ, Lipson MH, Graham JM Jr (1991). Radiological findings in Hallermann–Streiff syndrome: report of five cases and a review of the literature. Am J Med Genet 41:508–514

Cohen MM Jr (1991). Hallermann–Streiff syndrome: a review. Am J Med Genet 41:488–499

Dennis NR, Fairhurst J, Moore IE (1995). Lethal syndrome of slender bones, intrauterine fractures, characteristic facial appearance, and cataracts, resembling Hallerman-Streiff syndrome in two sibs. Am J Med Genet 59:517–520

Ollier Disease (see Enchondromatosis)

Omodysplasia [258315; 164745]

Clinical features: Variable shortening of the humeri and femora. Characteristic facies with a depressed nasal bridge and a long philtrum.

Radiographic features: Changes are maximal in the distal humerus, which is hypoplastic. The radial heads are dislocated anteriorly. Involvement of the femora is variable.

Genetics: AD; AR.

Other considerations: Although very rare, there is good evidence for the existence of mild AD and severe AR forms of the condition.

References:
Al Gazali LI, Al-Asaad FA (1995). Autosomal recessive omodysplasia. Clin Dysmorph 4:52–56

Baxova A, Maroteaux P, Barosova J, Netriova I (1994). Parental consanguinity in two sibs with omodysplasia. Am J Med Genet 49:263–265

Gugliantini P, Kozlowski K, Cappa M, Orazi C, Borrelli P, Pagnotta G (1991). Rhizomelic bone dysplasia with club-like femora. A distinctive, easily recognisable entity. La Radiologica Medica 81:550–552

Opsismodysplasia [258480]

Clinical features: Short-limbed rhizomelic dwarfism evident at birth, narrow thorax, depressed nasal bridge, hypotonia and susceptibility to respiratory infections. Death during the first decade.

Radiographic features: Ossification defect at the base of the skull. Gross platyspondyly with lack of vertebral ossification; short, thick, tubular bones with metaphyseal cupping and delayed epiphyseal ossification, square ilia, with horizontal acetabular roofs and medial and lateral spurs.

Genetics: AR.

Other considerations: Very rare.

References: Beemer FA, Kozlowski KS (1994). Additional case of opsismodysplasia supporting autosomal recessive inheritance. Am J Med Genet 49:344–347

Santos HG, Saraiva JM (1995). Opsismodysplasia: another case and literature review. Clin Dysmorph 4:222–226

Tyler K, Sarioglu N, Kunze J (1999). Five familial cases of opsismodysplasia substantiate the hypothesis of autosomal recessive inheritance. Am J Med Genet 83:47–52.

Oro-facial-digital Syndrome [311200; 258850]

Clinical features: Facial clefts, variable digital anomalies, including duplication or enlargement of the hallux; brachydactyly and syndactyly.

Radiographic features: Large first metatarsal and phalanges of the first toe, tarsal malformation, other inconsistent abnormalities in the hands and feet.

Genetics: Type I, X-linked dominant, with male lethality. Type II-VIII, AR.

Other considerations: The eponyms "Papillon-Léage" and "Mohr" have been used for types I and II, respectively.

References: Anneren G, Arvidson B, Gustavson K-H, Jorulf H, Carlsson G (1984). Oro-facial-digital syndromes I and II: radiological methods for diagnosis and the clinical variations. Clin Genet 26:178–186

Figuera LE, Rivas F, Cantu JM (1993). Oral-facial-digital syndrome with fibular aplasia: a new variant. Clin Genet 44:190–192

Fujiwara I, Kondo Y, Iinuma K (1999). Oral-facial-digital syndrome with hypothalamic hamartoma, postaxial ray hypoplasia of the limbs, and vagino-cystic communication: a new variant? Am J Med Genet 83:77–81

Toriello HV, Carey JC, Suslak E, Desposito FR, Leonard B, Lipson M, Friedman BD, Hoyme HE (1997). Six patients with oral-facial-digital

syndrome IV: the case for heterogeneity. Am J
Med Genet 69:250–260

OSMED (see Otospondylomegaepiphyseal Dysplasia) [215150]

Osteodysplastic Primordial Dwarfism (see Seckel Syndrome)

Osteodysplasty (Melnick–Needles Syndrome) [309350; 249420]

Clinical features: Characteristic facies with bulging eyes and a small
mandible, bowing of limbs, broad thumbs, vari-
able spinal malalignment.

Radiographic features: Irregular contours of the long bones and ribs,
"wavy" configuration of the tibia, metaphyseal
hypotubulation, supra-acetabular constriction of
the iliac bones, sclerosis of the base of the skull,
retarded skull ossification.

Genetics: XL with male lethality? AR form? (heterogeneous?).

Other considerations: The syndromic status of osteodysplasty remains
uncertain. An early onset AR from is termed "ter
Haar dysplasia".

References: Gorlin RJ, Langer LO (1978). Melnick–Needles
syndrome: radiographic alterations in the
mandible. Radiology 128:351–356
Krajewska-Walasek M, Winkielman J, Gorlin RJ
(1987). Melnick–Needles syndrome in males.
Am J Med Genet 27:153–158
Majewski F, Enders H, Ranke MB, Voit T (1993).
Serpentine fibula-polycystic kidney syndrome
and Melnick–Needles syndrome are different
disorders. Eur J Pediatr 152:916–921

Osteoectasia with Hyperphosphatasia (Juvenile Paget Disease) [239000]

Clinical features: Short stature, large skull, bowing of the long
bones, fractures, elevated serum alkaline phos-
phatase.

Radiographic features: Widening of all the bones with abnormal
trabecular pattern, bowing of the long bones,

cranial hyperostosis with patchy areas of sclerosis and lucency ("cotton-wool balls").

Genetics: AR.

Other considerations: About 30 reported cases. Skeletal changes resemble those of adult Paget disease, in severe degree.

References: Caffey J (1973). Familial hyperphosphatasemia with ateliosis and hypermetabolism of growing membranous bone: review of the clinical, radiographic and chemical features. Prog Pediatr Radiol 4:438–468

Spindler A, Berman A, Mautalen C, Ubios J, Santini AE (1992). Chronic idiopathic hyperphosphatasia: report of a case treated with pamidronate and a review of the literature. J Rheum 19:642–645

Whalen JP, Horwith M, Krook L, MacIntyre I, Mena E, Viteri F, Torun B, Nunez EA (1977). Calcitonin treatment in hereditary bone dysplasia with hyperphosphatasemia: a radiographic and histologic study of bone. Am J Roentgenol 129:29–35

Osteofibrous Dysplasia of the Tibia and Fibula (Campanacci Syndrome)

Clinical features: Anterolateral bowing of the shins.

Radiographic features: Enlargement and bowing of the tibia with irregular intracortical osteolytic and sclerotic changes.

Genetics: AR (?).

Other considerations: This disorder is probably fairly common and enters into the differential diagnosis of any obscure form of bowlegs.

References: Campanacci M, Laus M (1981). Osteofibrous dysplasia of the tibia and fibula. J Bone Joint Surg [Am] 63:367–371

Osteogenesis Imperfecta Group of Disorders

Osteogenesis Imperfecta (OI) was conventionally categorised into the Congenita form, which was evident at birth and the Tarda form, which presented in later childhood. With advances in knowledge, this sub-division has been superseded by a more complex numerical classification.

OI-I (corresponds to the former OI tarda). AD.   Common.
OI-II (corresponds to the former OI congenita).

	OI-IIa		AD, new mutation.	Common.
	OI-IIb		AR.	Rare.
	OI-IIc		AR.	Rare.
OI-III			AR/AD.	Uncommon.
OI-IV			AD.	Uncommon.

Further sub-division of OI-I and OI-IV on a basis of the presence or absence of tooth involvement (dentinogenesis imperfecta), has been proposed, but there is doubt concerning the validity of this concept. Sporadic unclassifiable examples of OI are not infrequent and there is debate as to whether or not many of them should be regarded as having OI-IV.

Other conditions, which have features in common with OI, include Bruck syndrome [259450] (OI with Congenital Contractures) and the Osteoporo-sis Pseudoglioma syndrome [259700].

Osteogenesis Imperfecta Tarda (OI-I, Several Forms) [166220; 166240]

Clinical features: Deformities of the long bones with tendency to fractures, wide bitemporal diameter, blue sclerae, sometimes dentinogenesis imperfecta, ligamentous hyperlaxity. Considerable variation in severity.

Radiographic features: The skeleton is usually gracile and porotic but the changes range from virtual normality to severe deformity. Multiple Wormian bones are always present and the sequelae of fractures may be evident.

Genetics: AD.

Other considerations: OI-I is common and heterogeneity is increasingly being recognised. Wormian bones are of diagnostic significance in doubtful cases. Bone fragility is a component of several rare familial disorders, including that documented by Nishimura et al (1999).

References:	Anderson PE Jr, Hauge M (1989). Osteogenesis imperfecta: a genetic, radiological, and epidemiological study. Clin Genet 36:250–255
	Nishimura G, Haga N, Aoki K, Hamazaki M, Tanigushi K, Iwaya T (1999). New brittle bone disorder: report of a family with six affected individuals. Am J Med Genet 84:320–329
	Willing MC, Pruchno CJ, Byers PH (1993). Molecular heterogeneity in osteogenesis imperfecta type I. Am J Med Genet 45:223–227

Osteogenesis Imperfecta Congenita (OI-II, Several Forms) [166210; 259400]

Clinical features:	Neonatal dwarfism with bowed, deformed limbs. Caput membranaceum and blue sclerae in some instances.
Radiographic features:	Osteoporosis, retarded and deficient skull ossification, multiple fractures. The "thick bone variety" is usually lethal (AD new mutation), while the "thin bone variety" (AR) has a better prognosis.
Genetics:	Heterogeneous, AD new mutations are common. AR forms are rare.
Other considerations:	OI congenita (OI-II) is fairly common and radiographic diagnosis is not difficult. The majority of examples are sporadic and represent AD mutations. In the AR Cole–Carpenter syndrome [112240], neonatal bone fragility is associated with craniostenosis and a typical facies. Astley–Kendall dysplasia is another lethal AR disorder in which ossification is defective.
References:	Cole WG, Dalgleish R (1995). Perinatal lethal osteogenesis imperfecta. J Med Genet 32:284–289
	Elçioglu N, Hall CM (1998). A lethal skeletal dysplasia with features of chondrodysplasia punctata and osteogenesis imperfecta: an

example of Astley–Kendall dysplasia. Further delineation of a rare genetic disorder. J Med Genet 35:505–507

MacDermot KD, Buckley B, Van Someren V (1995). Osteopenia, abnormal dentition, hydrops fetalis and communicating hydrocephalus. Clin Genet 48:217–220

Sillence DO, Barlow KK, Garber AP, Hall JG, Rimoin DL (1984). Osteogenesis imperfecta type II: delineation of the phenotype with reference to genetic heterogeneity. Am J Med Genet 17:407–423

Spranger J Cremin B, Beighton P (1982). Osteogenesis imperfecta congenita. Skeletal Radiol 8:35–38

Osteogenesis Imperfecta Type III [259420]

Clinical features: Severe fracturing tendency, stunted stature, white sclerae, variable dental involvement.

Radiographic features: Widespread bone deformity due to fracturing and malleability. "Wine-glass" pelvis, with severe protrusio acetabulae, Wormian bones in the cranial sutures.

Genetics: AR.

Other considerations: More than 100 affected persons have been identified in Southern Africa. OI III is uncommon in other populations. There is some confusion in the nosology, which has been expanded to include an AD form.

References:
Beighton P, Versfeld GA (1985). On the paradoxically high relative prevalence of osteogenesis imperfecta type III in the black population of South Africa. Clin Genet 27:398–401

Sillence DO, Barlow KK, Cole WG, Dietrich S, Garber AP, Rimoin DL (1986). Osteogenesis imperfecta type III: delineation of the phenotype with reference to genetic heterogeneity. Am J Med Genet 23:821–832

Viljoen D, Beighton P (1987). Osteogenesis imperfecta type III: an ancient mutation in Africa? Am J Med Genet 27:907–912

Osteogenesis Imperfecta Type IV

Clinical features: Variable fracturing tendency. White sclerae.

Radiographic features: As in OI-I.

Genetics: AD.

Other considerations: There is controversy concerning the syndromic identity of OI-IV.

References: Sillence DO (1988). Osteogenesis imperfecta, nosology and genetics. Ann NY Acad Sci 543:1–15

Osteogenesis Imperfecta with Congenital Contractures (Bruck Syndrome) [259450]

Clinical Features: Bone fragility and symmetrical contractions in the ankles and knees.

Radiographic Features: Skeletal lucency and gracility. Wormian bones in the cranial sutures.

Genetics: AR.

Other considerations: In the neonate the contractures often prompt an initial diagnosis of arthrogryposis multiplex congenita. The presence of Wormian bones in the skull clinches the diagnosis of Bruck syndrome.

References: Leroy JG, Nuytinck L, De Paepe A, De Rammelaere M, Gillerot Y, Verloes A, Loeys B, De Groote W (1998). Bruck syndrome: neonatal presentation and natural course in three patients. Pediatr Radiol 28:781–789
McPherson E, Clemens M (1997). Bruck syndrome (osteogenesis imperfecta with congenital joint contractures): review and report on the first North American case. Am J Med Genet 70:28–31
Viljoen D, Versfeld G, Beighton P (1989). Osteogenesis imperfecta with congenital joint contractures (Bruck syndrome). Clin Genet 36:122–126

Osteoglophonic Dysplasia [166250]

Clinical features: Rhizomelic dwarfism, severe facial abnormalities with frontal bossing, hypertelorism, and massive mandibular prognathism.

Radiographic features: Craniostenosis, fibrous dysplasia of the mandible, platyspondyly, and gross lucent defects in the metaphyses.

Genetics: Unknown.

Other considerations: Very rare, but unmistakable.

References: Beighton P, Cremin BJ, Kozlowski K (1980). Osteoglophonic dwarfism. Pediatr Radiol 10:46–50
Beighton P (1989). Osteoglophonic dysplasia. J Med Genet 26:572–576

Osteolysis Syndromes

The idiopathic osteolyses are a group of rare disorders characterised by progressive disappearance of bones. They are categorised in terms of the anatomical distribution of the abnormalities, with or without additional stigmata. When the changes are predominantly in the extremities, the designation "acro-osteolysis" is used; if the changes are widespread the terms "multicentric" or "generalised" are employed. It is noteworthy that there is considerable overlap between these disorders, and precise differentiation is not always possible.

1. Acro-osteolysis Syndromes

1.1 Phalangeal Acro-osteolysis [10.400;201300]

Clinical features: Shortening, deformity, dislocation of the terminal phalanges, abnormal nails.

Radiographic features: Osteolysis of the distal phalanges, progressing proximally.

Genetics: AD, AR (heterogeneous).

Other considerations: This condition must be distinguished from acquired disorders, notably vinyl chloride poisoning.

References: Brown DM, Bradford DS, Gorlin RJ, Desnick RJ, Langer LO Jr, Jowsey J, Sauk JJ Jr (1976). The

acro-osteolysis syndrome. Morphologic and
biochemical studies. J Pediatr 88:573–580
Harris DK and Adams WGF (1967) Acro-osteolysis occurring in men engaged in the polym-
erization of vinyl chloride. Br Med J 3:712–714
Kozlowski K, Barylak A, Eftekhari F, Pasyk K,
Wislocka E (1979). Acro-osteolysis. Problems
of diagnosis. Report of 4 cases. Pediatr Radiol
8:79–86

1.2 Phalangeal osteolysis, Hajdu–Cheney Type [102500]

Clinical features:
Hypermobile joints, abnormal skull, premature
loss of teeth. Polycystic kidneys are sometimes a
component.

Radiographic features:
Osteoporosis, fractures, distal phalangeal osteolysis, Wormian bones in the cranial sutures.

Genetics:
AD.

References:
Fryns J-P, Stinckens C, Feenstra L (1997). Vocal
cord paralysis and cystic kidney disease in
Hadju-Cheney syndrome. Clin Genet 51:271–
274
Kawamura J, Miki Y, Yamazaki S, Ogawa M
(1991). Hajdu–Cheney syndrome: MR imaging.
Neuroradiology 33:441–442.
O'Reilly MAR, Shaw DG (1994). Hadju-Cheney
syndrome. Ann Rheum Dis 53:276–279
Udell J, Schumacher JR, Kaplan F, Fallon MD
(1986). Idiopathic familial acroosteolysis: his-
tomorphometric study and literature review of
the Hajdu–Cheney syndrome. Arthritis Rheum
29:1032–1038

1.3 Carpotarsal Acro-osteolysis with and without nephropathy [166300]

Clinical features:
Shortening, deformity and limited movements in
the carpal and tarsal areas.

Radiographic features:
Progressive osteolysis of the carpal and tarsal
bones. Sometimes multicentric.

Genetics:
AD.

Other considerations:
Nephropathy is an important syndromic component in some affected families, but not in others.

References: Carnevale A, Canun S, Mendoza L, Castillo V del
                                  (1987). Idiopathic multicentric osteolysis with
                                  facial anomalies and nephropathy. Am J Med
                                  Genet 26:877–886
                                  Hardegger F, Simpson LA, Segmueller G (1985).
                                  The syndrome of idiopathic osteolysis: classi-
                                  fication, review, and case report. J Bone Joint
                                  Surg 67B:89–93
                                  Kozlowski K, Hanicka M, Garapich M (1971).
                                  Neurogene ulcerierende Akropathie (Akroos-
                                  teolyse Syndrom) Mschr Kinderheilk 119:1699–
                                  175
                                  Pai GS, Macpherson RI (1988). Idiopathic multi-
                                  centric osteolysis: report of two new cases and
                                  a review of the literature. Am J Med Genet
                                  29:929–936

1.4   Carpotarsal osteolysis, Francois Type *(Dermato-corneal dystrophy)* **[221800]**

Clinical features: Deformity of the hands, corneal opacities, skin
                                  xanthomata.

Radiographic features: Carpometacarpal and tarsometatarsal osteolysis.

Genetics: AR.

References: Bierly JR, George SP, Volpicelli M (1992).
                                  Dermochondroal corneal dystrophy (of Fran-
                                  cois). Br J Ophthal 76:760–761
                                  Caputo R, Sambvani B, Monti M, Caviccini S,
                                  Carassi A, Ratiglia A (1988). Dermochondro-
                                  corneal dystrophy (Francois syndrome): report
                                  of a case. Arch Dermatol 124:424–428

2.   Multicentric or Generalised Osteolysis Syndromes

2.1   Multicentric osteolysis, Torg Type *[259600;259610]*

Clinical features: Limitation of articular movements, subcutaneous
                                  nodules, fusiform digits.

Radiographic features: Osteoporosis, multicentric osteolysis with carpal,
                                  tarsal and interphalangeal involvement.

Genetics: AR.

References: Petit P, Fryns J-P (1986). Distal osteolysis, short
                                  stature, mental retardation, and characteristic
                                  facial appearance: delineation of an autosomal

recessive subtype of essential osteolysis. Am J
Med Genet 25:37-541

Torg JS, Digeorge AM, Kirkpatrick JA Jr, Trujillo
MM (1969). Hereditary multicentric osteolysis
with recessive transmission: a new syndrome. J
Pediatr 75:243-252.

2.2 Multicentric osteolysis, (mandibulo-acral dysplasia) [248370]

Clinical features: Short stature, bilateral clavicular hypoplasia,
dental crowding, stiff joints, atrophy of skin of
hands and feet, alopecia.

Radiographic features: Osteolysis of the phalanges, hypoplastic clavicles.

Genetics: AR.

Other considerations: Resembles progeria and cleido-cranial dysplasia.

References: Tenconi R, Miotti F, Miotti A, Audino G, Ferro R,
Clementi M (1986). Another Italian family with
mandibuloacral dysplasia: why does it seem
more frequent in Italy? Am J Med Genet
24:357-364.

Toriello HV (1995). Mandibulo-acral dysplasia:
Heterogeneity versus variability. Clin Dysmorph 4:12-24

2.3 Multicentric osteolysis, Winchester type [277950]

Clinical features: Short stature, marked joint contractures, corneal
opacities, coarse facies.

Radiographic features: Osteolysis of the carpus and tarsus, generalised
osteoporosis.

Genetics: AR.

General considerations: The clinical manifestations resemble rheumatoid
arthritis. There is some evidence that the muco-
polysaccharide metabolism is faulty.

References: Winchester P, Grossman H, Lim WN, Danes BS
(1969). A new acid mucopolysaccharidosis with
skeletal deformities simulating rheumatoid
arthritis. Am J Roentgenol 106:121-128.

Winter RM (1989). Winchester's syndrome. J Med
Genet 26:772-775

2.4 Familial expansile osteolysis *(Polyostotic Osteolytic Dysplasia) [174810]*

Clinical features:	Bone pain, pathological fractures, painful deformities, deafness, dental abnormalities. Onset in childhood.
Radiographic features:	Focal changes in the tubular bones which resemble those of Paget disease.
Genetics:	AD.
Other considerations:	The condition has been recognised in more than 40 persons in a family in Northern Ireland.
References:	Hughes AE, Shearman AM, Weber JL, Barr RJ, Wallace RGH, Osterberg PH, Nevin NC, Mollan RAB (1994). Genetic linkage of familial expansile osteolysis to chromosome 18q. Hum Molec Genet 3:359–361
	Osterberg PH, Wallace RGH, Adams DA, Crone RS, Dickson GR, Kanis JA, Mollan RAB, Nevin NC, Sloan J, Toner PG (1988). Familial expansile osteolysis: a new dysplasia. J Bone Joint Surg 70:255–260
	Wallace RGH, Barr RJ, Osterberg PH, Mollan RAB (1989). Familial expansile osteolysis. Clin Orthop Rel Res 248:265–277

2.5 Cystic Angiomatosis of Bone *(Gorham-Stout disease) [123880]*

Clinical Features:	Deformity due to cystic angiomatosis of bone. Sometimes asymptomatic.
Radiological Features:	Cystic osteolytic lesions in the long bones. Sclerotic obliteration with ageing.
Genetics:	AD, very rare.
Other considerations:	There is nosological confusion with Gorham osteolysis, which is a non-genetic disorder.
References:	Reid AB, Reid IL, Johnson G, Hamonic M, Major P (1989). Familial diffuse cystic angiomatosis of bone. Clin Orthop 238:211–218

2.6 Gorham Osteolysis *(monocentric massive osteolysis)*

Clinical features:	Localised deformity, often following trauma.
Radiographic features:	Progressive vanishing of bone. The thorax and pelvis are most often affected.

Genetics: Not hereditary.

Other considerations: This condition differs from cystic angiomatosis of bone (Gorham Stout disease) which is an AD trait [123880].

References: Choma ND, Biscotti CV, Bauer TW, Mehta AG, Licata AA (1987). Gorham's syndrome: A case report and review of the literature. Am J Med 83:1151–1156

Gorham LW, Stout AP (1955). Massive osteolysis (acute spontaneous absorption of bone, phantom bone, disappearing bone): its relation to hemangiomatosis. J Bone Joint Surg 37A:985–1004

Joseph J, Bartel E (1987). Disappearing bone disease: A case report and review of the literature. J Pediatr Orthop 7:584–588

Spieth ME, Greenspan A, Forrester DM, Ansari AN, Kimura RL, Gleason-Jordan I (1997). Gorham's disease of the radius: radiographic, scintographic, and MRI findings with pathologic correlation. Skeletal Radiol 26:659–663

Osteomesopycnosis (Osteomesopyknosis) [166450]

Clinical features: Spinal pains in adolescence or early adulthood.

Radiographic features: Sclerosis of the vertebral end-plates and pelvis. The proximal femora show cyst-like lesions, but the remaining bones are unaffected.

Genetics: AD.

Other considerations: Rare.

References: Maroteaux P (1980). L'Osteomésopycnose. Arch Fr Pediatr 37:153–158

Proschek R, Labelle H, Bard C, Marton D (1985). Osteomesopyknosis. Case report. J Bone Joint Surg (Am) 67A:652–653

Osteo-onychodysplasia (see Nail-Patella Syndrome)

Osteopathia Striata

Clinical features: Asymptomatic.

Radiographic features:	Linear striations at the ends of the tubular bones and in the iliac bones.
Genetics:	AD.
Other considerations:	Linear striations may be present in osteopetrosis and other sclerosing bone dysplasias, with Focal Dermal Hypoplasia [305600], in association with cranial sclerosis [166500] and with Hyperostosis Generalisata.
References:	Fujimoto H, Nishimura G, Tsumurai Y, Nosaka K, Kanisawa S, Ohba S, Tanaka Y (1999). Hyperostosis generalisata with striations of the bones: report of a female case and a review of the literature. Skeletal Radiol 28:460–464
	Gehweiler JA Bland WR, Carden TS, Daffner RH (1973). Osteopathia striata (Voorhoeve's disease); review of the roentgen manifestations. Am J Roentgenol 118:450–455
	Hurt RL (1953). Osteopathia striata: Voorhoeve's disease. J Bone Joint Surg [Br] 35:89–94

Osteopathia Striata with Cranial Sclerosis [166500]

Clinical features:	May be asymptomatic or present with macrocranium, facial palsy, and deafness. Cleft palate and mandibular hypoplasia may occur.
Radiographic features:	Sclerosis of the base of the skull, linear striations in the long bones.
Genetics:	AD?
Other considerations:	The disorder is probably underdiagnosed. Severity is variable and differentiation from uncomplicated osteopathia striata may not be easy. In the putative XL form, affected males with multiple congenital anomalies may be stillborn.
References:	Horan FT, Beighton PG (1978). Osteopathia striata with cranial sclerosis. An autosomal dominant entity. Clin Genet 13:201–206
	Konig R, Dukiet C, Dorries A, Zabel B, Fuchs S (1996). Osteopathia striata with cranial sclerosis: variable expressivity in a four generation pedigree. Am J Med Genet 63:68–73

Pellegrino JE, McDonald-McGinn DM, Schneider A, Markowitz RI, Zackai EH (1997). Further clinical delineation and increased morbidity in males with osteopathia striata with cranial sclerosis: an X-linked disorder? Am J Med Genet 70:159–165

Savarirayan R, Nance J, Morris L, Haan E, Couper R (1997). Osteopathia striata with cranial sclerosis: highly variable phenotypic expression within a family. Clin Genet 52:199–205

Osteopetroses

The osteopetroses, also known as "stony bones", or "marble bones" are a group of skeletal dysplasias characterised by increased radiological density of bone. These have been conventionally sub-divided into the benign or delayed AD form and the malignant, precocious or lethal AR form. More recently, other varieties have been delineated, and the following are now recognised.

Osteopetrosis with Delayed Manifestations	AD
Osteopetrosis with Precocious Manifestations	AR
Osteopetrosis, Intermediate type	AR
Osteopetrosis, with Renal Tubular Acidosis	AR

The term "Albers–Schönberg disease", has been used loosely for any sclerosing bone dysplasia, but in its precise sense, the eponym is applicable to AD osteopetrosis with delayed manifestations.

Osteopetrosis with Delayed Manifestations (Benign Osteopetrosis) [166000]

Clinical features: May be asymptomatic or present with anaemia, fractures, compression of the 7th or 8th cranial nerves or with osteomyelitis of the mandible.

Radiographic features: Generalised osteosclerosis, most evident in the skull. Variable hypotubulation of the long bones with linear striations and transverse bands. Vertebral sclerosis ("rugger jersey" spine).

Genetics: AD, heterogeneous.

Other considerations: Sub-division into Types I and II on a basis of the presence or absence of transverse vertebral sclerosis has been made and a Type III has been proposed.

References:

Cooper JR, Sprigg A (1998). Slipped capital femoral epiphysis in a patient with type II autosomal dominant osteopetrosis. Skeletal Radiol 27:515–517

El-Tawil T, Stoker DJ (1993). Benign osteopetrosis: a review of 42 cases showing two different patterns. Skel Radiol 22:587–593

Lund-Sørensen N, Gudmundsen TE, Østensen H (1997). Autosomal dominant osteopetrosis: report of a Norwegian family with radiographic or anamnestic findings differing from the generally accepted classification. Skeletal Radiol 26:173–176

Takacs I, Cooper H, Weaver DD, Econs MJ (1999). Bone mineral density and laboratory evaluation of a Type II autosomal dominant osteopetrosis carrier. Am J Med Genet 85:9–12

Osteopetrosis with Precocious Manifestations (Malignant or Infantile Osteopetrosis [259700]

Clinical features: Failure to thrive in infancy, hepatosplenomegaly, anaemia. Potentially lethal.

Radiographic features: Progressive generalised osteosclerosis. Marked expansion of metaphyses of the long bones with "endobones" and transverse bands of decreased and increased density.

Genetics: AR.

Other considerations: Rare. May respond to bone marrow transplantation or treatment with interferon. Other rare osteosclerotic disorders that are lethal in the neonate include Blomstrand dysplasia [215045] and Raine dysplasia [259775].

References:

Bollerslev J (1987). Osteopetrosis: a genetic and epidemiological study. Clin Genet 31:86–90

Brodie SG, Lachman RS, McGovern MM, Mekikian PB, Wilcox WR (1999). Lethal osteosclerotic skeletal dysplasia with intracellular inclusion bodies. Am J Med Genet 83:372–377

Fiscjer A, Friedrich W, Levinsky R, Vossen J, Griscelli C, Kubanek B, Morgan G, Wagemaker G, Landais P (1986). Bone marrow transplantation for immunodeficiencies and osteopetrosis: European survey, 1958–1985. Lancet II:1080–1084

Key LL Jr, Rodriguiz RM, Willi SM, Wright NM, Hatcher HC, Eyre DR, Cure JK, Griffin PP, Ries WL (1995). Long-term treatment of osteopetrosis with recombinant human interferon gamma. New Eng J Med 332:1594–1599

Loriá-Cortés R, Quesada-Calvo E, Cordero-Chaverri C (1977). Osteopetrosis in children: A report of 26 cases. J Pediatr 91:43–47

Osteopetrosis, Intermediate Form [259710]

Clinical features: As benign AD osteopetrosis [166000]. Greater tendency to fracturing and osteomyelitis of the jaw.

Radiographic features: As benign osteopetrosis.

Genetics: AR.

Other considerations: It is difficult to distinguish an isolated case from benign osteopetrosis.

References: Beighton P, Horan F, Hamersma H (1977). A review of the osteopetroses. Postgrad Med J 53:507–517

Kahler SG, Burns JA, Aylsworth AS (1984). A mild autosomal recessive form of osteopetrosis. Am J Med Genet 17:451–464

Kaibari N, Katsuki I, Hotokebuchi T, Takagishi K (1982). Intermediate form of osteopetrosis with recessive inheritance. Skeletal Radiol 9:47–51

Osteopetrosis with Renal Tubular Acidosis and Carbonic Anhydrase II Deficiency [259730]

Clinical features: Onset in childhood with failure to thrive and renal tubular acidosis.

Radiographic features: As for benign AD osteopetrosis [166000] with additional intracranial calcification.

Genetics: AR, heterogeneous.

Other consideration: The diagnosis is confirmed by demonstration of defective activity of carbonic anhydrase II in red blood cells. High frequency in Saudi Arabia.

References: Ohlsson A, Cumming WA, Paul A, Sly WS (1986). Carbonic anhydrase II deficiency syndrome: recessive osteopetrosis with renal tubular acidosis and cerebral calcification. Pediatrics 77:371–381

Sly WS, Whyte MP, Sundaram V, Tashian RE, Hewett-Emmett D, Guibaud P, Vainsel M, Baluarte HJ, Gruskin A, Al-Mosawi M, Sakati N, Ohlsson A (1985). Carbonic anhydrase II deficiency in 12 families with the autosomal recessive syndrome of osteopetrosis with renal tubular acidosis and cerebral calcification. New Eng J Med 313:139–145

Strisciuglio P, Sartorio R, Pecoraro C, Lotito F, Sly WS (1990). Variable clinical presentation of carbonic anhydrase deficiency: evidence for heterogeneity? Europ J Pediat 149:337–340

Osteopoikilosis (Buschke–Ollendorff Syndrome) [166700]

Clinical features: Asymptomatic, usually a chance diagnosis. Skin changes (dermatofibrosis lenticularis disseminata) are inconspicuous.

Radiographic features: Multiple small, round, sclerotic foci at the ends of the long bones and in the pelvis.

Genetics: AD.

Other considerations: The main importance of osteopoikilosis lies in the differentiation from multiple secondary neoplastic deposits. A variety of minor malformations may coexist.

References: Gunal I, Seber S, Basaran N, Artan S, Gunal K, Gokturk E (1993). Dacryocystitis associated with osteopoikilosis. Clin Genet 44:211–213

Langier R, Mbakop A, Bigler A (1984). Osteopoikilosis: A radiological and pathological study. Skeletal Radiol 11:161–168

Sarralde A, Garcia-Cruz D, Nazara Z, Sanchez-Corona J (1994). Osteopoikilosis: report of a familial case. Genet Counsel 5:373–375

Osteoporosis (see Juvenile Idiopathic Osteoporosis)

Osteoporosis-Pseudoglioma Syndrome [259770]

Clinical features:	Ocular pseudogliomata, retinal detachment, bone fragility leading to multiple fractures and variable mild mental retardation.
Radiographic features:	Osteoporosis, fractures, Wormian bones.
Genetics:	AR.
Other considerations:	The skeletal changes mimic osteogenesis imperfecta. The eye abnormalities are a pointer to the correct diagnosis.
References:	De Paepe A, Leroy JG, Nuytinck L, Meire F, Capoen J (1993). Osteoporosis-pseudoglioma syndrome. Am J Med Genet 45:30–37
	Frontali M, Stomea C, Dallapiccola B (1985). Osteoporosis-pseudoglioma syndrome: report of three affected sibs and an overview. Am J Med Genet 22:35–47
	Somer H, Palotie A, Somer M, Hoikka V, Peltonen L (1988). Osteoporosis-pseudoglioma syndrome: Clinical, morphological and biochemical studies. J Med Genet 25:543–549

Osteosclerosis, Stanescu type (Craniofacial Dysostosis with Diaphyseal Hyperplasia) [122900]

Clinical features:	Short stature, rhizomelia, brachydactyly, characteristic small facies with pointed nose, dental abnormalities.
Radiographic features:	Widening and sclerosis of the cortices of the long bones, small sinuses, obtuse mandibular angle, brachydactyly.
Genetics:	AD.

Other considerations: This disorder must be distinguished from other AR osteoscleroses in which the hair is involved, notably osteosclerosis with bamboo hair (Netherton syndrome) [256500] and Tricho-thiodystrophy [242170]. The AD Trichodentoosseous syndrome [190320], in which mild bone density is associated with hair and tooth abnormalities, also enters into the differential diagnosis. Neonatal bone sclerosis is a major manifestation of rare AR conditions, notably Blomstrand chondrodysplasia [215045] and Raine lethal osteosclerosis [259775].

References: Dipierri JE, Gutman JD (1984). A second family with autosomal dominant osteosclerosis – type Stanescu. Am J Med Genet 18:13–18

Happle R, Traupe H, Grobe H, Bonsmann G (1984). The Tay syndrome (congenital ichthyosis with trichothiodystrophy). Eur J Pediatr 141:147–152.

Horovitz DDG, Neto JGB, Boy R, Vargas FR, Llerena JC Jr, Cabral de Almeida JC (1995). Autosomal dominant osteosclerosis type Stanescu: the third family. Am J Med Genet 57:605–609

Kan AE, Kozlowski K (1992). New distinct lethal osteosclerotic bone dysplasia (Raine syndrome). Am J Med Genet 43:860–864

Price JA, Wright JT, Walker SJ, Crawford PJM, Aldred MJ, Hart TC (1999). Tricho-dento-osseous syndrome and amelogenesis imperfecta with taurodontism are genetically distinct conditions. Clin Genet 56:35–40

Young ID, Zuccullo JM, Broderick NJ (1993). A lethal skeletal dysplasia with generalised sclerosis and advanced skeletal maturation: Blomstrand chondrodysplasia? J Med Genet 30:155–157

Oto-palato-digital Syndrome (OPDI) [311300]

Clinical features: Short stature, conductive deafness, cleft palate, broad short hallux and thumb, distinctive facies. Dental abnormalities. Females are much less severely affected than males.

Radiographic features: Hand and foot abnormalities – short distal phalanges, fused and supernumerary carpal and tarsal bones, wide vertebral interpediculate distances, high iliac angles, large cranium.

Genetics: XL, with partial manifestation in carrier females.

Other considerations: OPDII [304120] is a similar, but more severe disorder in which mental retardation is an additional component.

References: Kozlowski K, Turner G, Scougall J, Harrington J (1977). Oto-palato-digital syndrome with severe x-ray changes in two half brothers. Pediatr Radiol 6:97–102

Pazzaglia UE, Beluffi G (1986). Oto-palato-digital syndrome in four generations of a large family. Clin Genet 30:338–344

Superti-Furga A, Gimelli F (1987). Fronto-metaphyseal dysplasia and the otopalato-digital syndrome. Dysmorph Clin Genet 1:2–5

Oto-spondylo-megaepiphyseal Dysplasia (OSMED) [215150]

Clinical features: Stunted stature, depressed nasal bridge, severe progressive deafness, cleft palate.

Radiographic features: Abnormally large epiphyses, platyspondyly and progressive fusion of carpal bones.

Genetics: AR.

Other considerations: This condition is also known as chondrodystrophy with sensorineural deafness, osteomegaepiphyseal dysplasia, Nance-Sweeney dysplasia and the Nance-Insley syndrome. A form in which osteoporosis is a major feature may be an autonomous entity. The round femoral inferior epiphyseal type of recessive chondrodysplasia is a similar disorder.

References: Giedion A, Brandner M, Lecannellier J, Muhar U, Prader A, Sulzer J, Zweymüller E (1982). Oto-spondylo-megaepiphyseal dysplasia (OSMED). Helv Paediat Acta 37:361–380

McAlister W, Coe SD, Whyte MP (1986). Macro-epiphyseal dysplasia with symptomatic osteo-

porosis, wrinkled skin and aged appearance.
Skeletal Radiol 15:47–51

Rosser EM, Hall CM, Harper J, Lacour M,
Baraitser M (1996). Nance-Sweeney chondrodysplasia – a further case? Clin Dysmorph
5:207–212

Pachydermoperiostosis (Idiopathic Hypertrophic Osteoarthropathy) [167100]

Clinical features: Hypertrophy of the skin and soft tissues of the hands and feet with digital clubbing. Facial pachydermia. More severe in males.

Radiographic features: Periosteal thickening of the long bones.

Genetics: AD (AR form?)

Other considerations: A few variants have been reported. The dermal changes serve to distinguish the condition from pulmonary osteoarthropathy and thyroid acropathy.

References: Hedayati H, Barmada R, Skosey JL (1980). Acrolysis in pachydermoperiostosis (primary or idiopathic hypertrophic osteoarthropathy). Arch Intern Med 140:1087–1088

Joseph B, Chacko V (1985). Acro-osteolysis associated with hypertrophic pulmonary osteoarthropathy and pachydermoperiostosis. Radiology 154:343–344

Matucci-Cerinic M, Cinti S, Morroni M, Lotti T, Nuzzaci G, Lucebte E, di Lollo S, Ceruso M, Cagnoni M (1989). Pachydermoperiostosis (primary hypertrophic osteoarthropathy): report of a case with evidence of endothelial and connective tissue involvement. Ann Rheum Dis 48:240–246

Papillon-Léage Syndrome (see Oro-facial-digital Syndrome)

Parastremmatic Dysplasia [168400]

Clinical features:	Severe dwarfism, kyphoscoliosis, asymmetric deformities of the extremities, multiple joint contractures.
Radiographic features:	Diagnostic floccular appearance of the epiphyses and metaphyses. Small pelvis with irregular calcification. Retarded development of the femoral heads. Generalised osteoporosis.
Genetics:	AD (?). Very rare.
References:	Horan F, Beighton P (1976). Parastremmatic dwarfism. J Bone Joint Surg [Br] 58:343–347
	Langer LO, Petersen D, Spranger J (1970). An unusual bone dysplasia: parastremmatic dwarfism. Am J Roentgenol 110:550–560

Parenti-Fraccaro Type Achondrogenesis (see Achondrogenesis Type I)

Patellar Hypoplasia (Small Patella Syndrome) [168860]

Clinical features:	Absence or hypoplasia of the patella.
Radiographic features:	As above.
Genetics:	AD.
Other considerations:	Rare. Must be differentiated from nail-patella syndrome.
References:	Braun H-S (1978). Familial aplasia or hypoplasia of the patella. Clin Genet 13:350–352

Pena–Shokeir Syndrome (see Cerebro-oculo-facio-skeletal Syndrome)

Perthes Disease

Clinical features:	Hip pain and disturbed gait in childhood.

Radiographic features: Flattening and irregularity of the femoral capital epiphyses.

Genetics: Non-genetic.

Other considerations: Perthes disease is very common, but atypical or bilateral cases should always arouse suspicion of a genetic bone dysplasia syndrome, as many present with Perthes-like manifestations. In Meyer dysplasia, changes that are confined to the femoral heads resemble those of Perthes disease. The aetiology of this condition is uncertain.

References: Meyer J (1963). Dysplasia epiphysealis capitis femoris. Acta Orthop Scand 34:183–189
                          Wynne-Davies R, Gormley J (1978). The aetiology of Perthes disease. J Bone Joint Surg [Br] 60:6–14

Phocomelia (including the Roberts Pseudothalidomide Syndrome) [268300]

Clinical features: Malformed extremities articulate directly with the trunk. The anomalies may be asymmetrical and variable in degree.

Radiographic features: Variable hypoplasia or aplasia of the long bones.

Genetics: AR.

Other considerations: Thalidomide embryopathy is the classical cause of phocomelia, but this malformation is also a feature of the Roberts Syndrome. In this entity, an unusual facies, sparse hair, and visceral abnormalities are additional features. The pseudothalidomide, or SC syndrome may be the same disorder.

References: Fryns JP, Kleczkowska A, Moerman P, Van Den Berghe K, Van Den Berghe H (1987). The Roberts tetraphocomelia syndrome: identical limb defects in two siblings. Am J Med Genet 30:243–245
                          Romke C, Froster-Iskenius U, Heyne K, Hohn W, Hof M, Grzejszczyk G, Rauskolb R, Rehder H, Schwinger E (1987). Roberts syndrome and SC phocomelia: a single genetic entity. Clin Genet 31:170–177

Platyspondylic Lethal Dysplasia (see Spondylodysplasia)

Polycystic Osteodysplasia with Progressive Dementia

Clinical features:	Progressive dementia with onset in early adulthood, epilepsy.
Radiographic features:	Cystic changes in the carpus, tarsus and tubular bones of the extremities.
Genetics:	AR?
Other considerations:	Rare. Most cases reported from Finland.
References:	Hakola HPA, Iivanainen M (1973). A new hereditary disease with progressive dementia and polycystic osteodysplasia: neuroradiological analysis of seven cases. Neuroradiol 6:162–168

Polyostotic Fibrous Dysplasia (see Fibrous Dysplasia, Jaffe–Lichtenstein Syndrome)

Popliteal Pterygium Syndrome (see Multiple Pterygium Syndrome)

Primordial Dwarfism (see Seckel Syndrome)

Progeria [176670]

Clinical features:	Growth failure in infancy followed by precocious ageing, loss of subcutaneous fat, peculiar facies, and alopecia. Normal mental development.
Radiographic features:	Thin bones, coxa valga, clavicular hypoplasia, acro-osteolysis. Delayed ossification of the cranium, with multiple wormian bones.
Genetics:	Unknown. New AD mutation?
Other considerations:	Well defined. More than 100 known cases. The Wiedemann-Rautenstrauch neonatal progeroid syndrome is a separate AR entity [264090].
References:	Reichel W, Bailey JA II, Zigel S, Garcia-Brunel R, Knox G (1971). Radiological findings in progeria. J Am Geriatr Soc 19:657–674

Rodríguez JI, Pérez-Alonso P, Funes R, Pérez-Rodríguez J (1999). Lethal neonatal Hutchinson–Gilford progeria syndrome. Am J Med Genet 82:242–248

Toriello HV (1990). Wiedemann-Rautenstrauch syndrome. J Med Genet 27:256–257

Progressive Pseudorheumatoid Dysplasia [208230]

Clinical features: Childhood onset of a progressive arthropathy that resembles rheumatoid arthritis (RA), with swelling of digits, apparent enlargement of joints, stiffness and contractures. Investigations for classical RA are negative.

Radiographic features: Digits show narrow joint spaces with wide metaphyses and flat epiphyses. Femoral heads are enlarged and the acetabula are irregular. Platyspondyly with erosion of the anterior portions of the end-plates is present.

Genetics: AR.

Other considerations: This condition can mimic juvenile RA. The recurrence in siblings, negative RA investigations and the absence of periarticular erosions are pointers to the correct diagnosis.

References:

El-Shanti H, Omari HZ, Qubain HI (1997). Progressive pseudorheumatoid dysplasia: report of a family and review. J Med Genet 34:559–563

Kozlowski K, Kennedy J, Lewis IC (1986). Radiographic features of progressive pseudorheumatoid arthritis. Australas Radiol 30:244–250

Legius E, Mulier M, van Damme B, Fryns JP (1993). Progressive pseudorheumatoid arthritis of childhood (PPAC) and normal adult height. Clin Genet 44:152–156

Rezai-Delui H, Mamoori G, Sadri-Mahvelati E, Noori NM (1994). Progressive pseudorheumatoid chondrodysplasia: a report of nine cases in three families. Skeletal Radiol 23:411–419

Proteus Syndrome [176920]

Clinical features:	Asymmetrical overgrowth of the extremities, soft tissue hypertrophy, skin naevi, multiple benign osseous and subcutaneous tumours.
Radiographic features:	Osteomata, exostoses, localised hypertrophy.
Genetics:	Non-genetic?
Other considerations:	The condition must be differentiated from the Klippel–Trenaunay–Weber syndrome, Maffucci syndrome and encephalo-cranio-cutaneous lipomatosis.
References:	Biesecker LG, Happle R, Mulliken JB, Weksberg R, Graham JM Jr, Viljoen DL, Cohen MM Jr (1999). Proteus syndrome: diagnostic criteria, differential diagnosis, and patient evaluation. Am J Med Genet 84:389–395
	Gordon PL, Wilroy RS, Lasater OE, Cohen MM Jr (1995). Neoplasms in Proteus syndrome. Am J Med Genet 57:74–78
	Viljoen DL, Nelson MM, de Jong G, Beighton P (1987). Proteus syndrome in Southern Africa: natural history and clinical manifestations in six individuals. Am J Med Genet 27:87–97

Proximal Focal Femoral Dysplasia (see Femoral Facial Syndrome)

Pseudoachondroplasia [177150]

Clinical features:	Short-limb dwarfism. Normal head and face. Variable spinal malalignment. Lax stubby digits in some forms.
Radiographic features:	Vertebral involvement is variable, but tends to regress in adulthood. Long bones have small irregular epiphyses and uneven splayed metaphyses.
Genetics:	AD. Reported sibling pairs were probably the result of gonadal mosaicism rather than autosomal recessive inheritance.

Other considerations: Pseudoachondroplasia is a well recognised cause of dwarfism. The faulty gene is on chromosome 19 at the same locus as MED, Fairbank type [132400].

References: Heselson NG, Cremin B, Beighton P (1977). Pseudoachondroplasia: a report of 13 cases. Br J Radiol 50:473–482

Kozlowski K (1976). Pseudoachondroplastic dysplasia: a critical analysis. Australas Radiol 20:255–269

Marik I, Kozlowski K (1998). Severe pseudoachondroplasia in a mother and her son. Radiol Med 96:98–100

McKeans J, Rotta J, Hecht JT (1996). Natural history study of pseudoachondroplasia. Am J Med Genet 63:406–410

Pseudodiastrophic Dysplasia [264180]

Clinical features: Rhizomelic limb shortening, severe clubfoot, scoliosis, multiple dislocations of phalanges and a typical facies.

Radiographic features: Generalised involvement of the major skeletal components. Platyspondyly with anterior projection in the lumbar region. Increased bitemporal diameter.

Genetics: AR.

Other considerations: Resembles mild diastrophic dysplasia. Propensity to hyperthermia and to C1-C2 dislocation due to odontoid hypoplasia.

References: Eteson DJ, Beluffi G, Burgio GR, Belloni C, Lachman RS, Rimoin DL (1986). Pseudodiastrophic dysplasia: a distinct newborn skeletal dysplasia. J Pediat 109:635–641.

Pseudohypoparathyroidism (Albright Hereditary Osteodystrophy) [103580; 300800]

Clinical features: Short stature, obesity, mental retardation, round face, brachydactyly, corneal or lenticular opacities. Variable hypocalcaemia and hyperphosphataemia.

Radiographic features: Short metacarpals, particularly the 4th and 5th. Short distal phalanx of the thumb. Cone-shaped epiphyses. Subcutaneous and basal ganglia calcifications. Generalised coarse trabeculations, osteosclerosis or osteoporosis. Variable craniostenosis and exostoses.

Genetics: AD (?). XL dominant (?).

Other considerations: Pseudopseudohypoparathyroidism is the same disorder, without hypocalcaemia, and represents variation of a single genetic defect.

References: Fitch N (1982). Albright's hereditary osteodystrophy: A review. Am J Med Genet 11(1):11–29
Steinbach HL, Young DA (1968). The roentgen appearance of pseudohypoparathyroidism (PH) and pseudopseudohypoparathyroidism (PPH). Am J Roentgenol 97:49–55
Hewitt M, Chambers TL (1988). Early presentation of pseudohypoparathyroidism. J R Soc Med 81:666–667

Pseudopolydystrophy of Maroteaux (see Complex Carbohydrate Metabolic Disorders)

Pycnodysostosis [265800]

Clinical features: Short stature. Obtuse mandibular angle. Patent fontanelles. Fractures.

Radiographic features: Generalised osteosclerosis with normal bone modelling. Delayed skull ossification with wide fontanelles. Increased mandibular angle. Acroosteolysis. Fractures.

Genetics: AR.

Other considerations: Uncommon, but has wide geographic distribution. Variants have been reported.

References: Edelson JG, Obad S, Geiger R, On A, Artul HJ (1992). Pycnodysostosis: orthopedic aspects with a description of 14 new cases.

Mills KLG, Johnston AW (1988). Pycnodysostosis.
J Med Genet 25:550–553
Srivastava KK, Bhattacharya AK, Galatius-Jensen
F, Tamaela LA, Borgstein A, Kozlowski K
(1978). Pycnodysostosis (report of four cases).
Australas Radiol 22:70–76

Pyle Dysplasia (see Metaphyseal Dysplasia)

Radial Aplasia-Thrombocytopenia Syndrome (TAR Syndrome) [274000]

Clinical features: Malformed or absent radial ray bones. Thrombo-cytopenia develops in infancy.

Radiographic features: Radial hypoplasia, often associated with other limb deformities.

Genetics: AR.

Other considerations: Distinguished from Fanconi pancytopenia syndrome by the onset of haematological problems in infancy. There is some overlap with the Roberts Pseudothalidomide syndrome [268300].

References: Hall J (1987). Thrombocytopenia and absent radius (TAR) syndrome. J Med Genet 24:79–83
Schnur RE, Eunpu DL, Zackai EH (1987). Thrombocytopenia with absent radius in a boy and his uncle. Am J Med Genet 28:117–123
Urban M, Opitz C, Bommer C, Enders H, Tinschert S, Witkowski R (1998). Bilaterally cleft lip, limb defects, and haematological manifestations: Roberts syndrome versus TAR syndrome. Am J Med Genet 79:155–160

RAPADILINO Syndrome [266280]

Clinical features: Radial and patellar aplasia, with absence of thumbs, joint dislocations and an unusual facies.

Radiographic features: As above.

Genetics: AR.

Other considerations:	Rare. The majority of affected persons have been documented in Finland. The term "RAPADILINO" is an acronym, derived from the manifestations of the disorder.
References:	Kaariainen H, Ryoppy S, Norio R (1989). RAPADILINO syndrome with radial and patellar aplasia/hypoplasia as main manifestations. Am J Med Genet 33:346–351
	Vargas FR, Cabral de Almeida JC, Llerena JC Jr, Reis DF (1992). RAPADILINO syndrome. Am J Med Genet 44:716–719

Rheinhardt–Pfeiffer Type of Mesomelic Dysplasia (see Mesomelic Dysplasia)

Rickets, Hypophosphataemic and Other Forms [307800; 264700]

Clinical features:	Vitamin D-resistant, renal, and other forms of metabolic rickets share the common clinical features of skeletal distortion. The changes vary in severity from gross limb and spinal deformity to minor bowing of the legs.
Radiographic features:	The bones are lucent, with an altered trabecular pattern, and the metaphyses are irregular. Diagnostic distinction is by biochemical studies, as the radiographic stigmata are non-specific.
Genetics:	The common form of vitamin D-resistant rickets is inherited as an XL dominant, while the pseudovitamin-D deficiency, renal and metabolic types are autosomal recessive.
Other considerations:	The genetic metaphyseal chrondrodysplasias may present a similar appearance and lead to diagnostic confusion.
References	Burnet CH, Dent CE, Harper C, Warland BJ (1964). Vitamin D-resistant rickets. Analysis of twenty-four pedigrees with hereditary and sporadic cases. Am J Med 36:222–228
	Hardy DC, Murphy WA, Siegel BA, Reid IR, Whyte MP (1989). X-linked hypophosphatemia

in adults: prevalence of skeletal radiographic
and scintigraphic features. Radiology 171:403–
414

Scriver CR, Tenenhouse HS, Glorieux FH (1991).
X-linked hypophosphatemia: an appreciation
of a classic paper and a survey of progress since
1958. Medicine 70:218–228

Roberts Pseudothalidomide Syndrome (see Phocomelia)

Robinow Type of Mesomelic Dysplasia (see Mesomelic Dysplasia)

Rothmund–Thomson Syndrome [268400]

Clinical features: Small stature, dermal erythema, photosensitivity
and hyperkeratosis, mental retardation. Defective
nails and teeth, juvenile cataract. Distal limb
malformations.

Radiographic features: Hypoplasia of the thumb and radius. Generalised
osteoporosis, patchy sclerosis, and abnormal
trabeculation. Bone cysts. Subcutaneous calcification. Acro-osteolysis.

Genetics: AR.

Other considerations: More than 50 known cases. The striking stigmata
are unmistakable.

References: Hall JG, Pagon RA, Wilson KM (1980). Rothmund–Thomson syndrome with severe dwarf-
ism. Am J Dis Child 134:165–169

Lindor NM, Devries EMG, Michels VV, Schad CR,
Jalal SM, Donovan KM, Smithson WA, Kvols
LK, Thibodeau SN, Dewald GW (1996). Roth-
mund–Thomson syndrome in siblings: evi-
dence for acquired in vivo mosaicism. Clin
Genet 49:124–129

Maurer RM, Langford OL (1967). Rothmund's
syndrome. A cause of resorption of phalangeal
tufts and dystropic calcification. Radiology
89:706–807

Starr DG, McClure JP, Connor JM (1985). Non-
dermatological complications and genetic as-

pects of the Rothmund–Thomson syndrome.
Clin Genet 27:102–104

Rubinstein–Taybi Syndrome [180849]

Clinical features: Short stature, mental retardation, long bulbous beaked nose, broad thumbs.

Radiographic features: Enlarged terminal phalanges of the thumbs and great toes. Retarded bone age. Occasional stippling of the femoral capital epiphyses. Other variable non-diagnostic skeletal abnormalities.

Genetics: Microdeletion?

Other considerations: A well-defined mental retardation syndrome.

References: Bonioli E, Bellini C, Sénès FM, Palmieri A, Di Stadio M, Pinelli G (1993). Slipped capital femoral epiphysis associated with Rubinstein–Taybi syndrome. Clin Genet 44(2):79–81
Stevens CA, Carey JC, Blackburn BL (1990). Rubinstein–Taybi syndrome: a natural history study. Am J Med Genet Suppl 6:30–37
Wallerstein R, Anderson CE, Hay B, Gupta P, Gibas L, Ansari K, Cowchock FS, Weinblatt V, Reid C, Levitas A, Jackson L (1997). Submicroscopic deletions at 16p133.3 in Rubinstein–Taybi syndrome: frequency and clinical manifestations in a North American population. J Med Genet 34:203–206

Russell–Silver Syndrome [180860]

Clinical features: Low birth weight, small stature, asymmetry usually of the limbs, triangular facies, café-au-lait spots.

Radiographic features: Asymmetry, retarded bone age, minor vertebral abnormalities.

Genetics: AD, new mutation? Microdeletion?

Other considerations: Separate syndromic status of the Russell and the Silver syndromes has been proposed but remains unconfirmed.

References: Duncan PA, Hall JG, Shapiro LR, Vibert BK
                                (1990). Three-generation dominant trans-
                                mission of the Silver-Russell syndrome. Am J
                                Med Genet 35:245–250
                                Herman TE, Crawford JD, Cleveland RH, Kushner
                                DC (1987). Hand radiographs in Russell–Silver
                                syndrome. Pediatrics 79:743–744
                                Patton MA (1988). Russell–Silver syndrome. J
                                Med Genet 25:557–560
                                Preece MA, Price SM, Davies V, Clough L, Stanier
                                P, Trembath RC, Moore GE (1997). Maternal
                                uniparental disomy 7 in Silver-Russell syn-
                                drome. J Med Genet 34:609

Saldino–Mainzer Dysplasia (Acrodysplasia with Retinitis Pigmentosa and Nephropathy) [266920]

Clinical features: Stubby digits, stunted stature, retinitis pigmento-
                                sa and renal abnormalities.

Radiographic features: Phalangeal shortening, indistinguishable from the
                                acrodysplasias.

Genetics: AR?, rare.

Other considerations: Hereditary renal-retinal dysplasia is an alternative
                                designation. There is some doubt about the
                                autonomous syndromic status of this disorder.

References: Giedion A (1979). Phalangeal cone-shaped epi-
                                physes of the hands and chronic renal failure.
                                The conorenal syndrome. Pediatr Radiol 8:32–38
                                Mendley SR, Poznanski AK, Spargo BH, Langman
                                CB (1995). Hereditary sclerosing glomerulo-
                                pathy in the conorenal syndrome. Am J Kidney
                                Dis 25:792–797
                                Saldino RM, Mainzer F (1971). Cone-shaped
                                epiphyses in siblings with hereditary renal
                                disease and retinitis pigmentosa. Radiology
                                98:39–45

Saldino–Noonan Syndrome (see Short Rib Syndrome type I)

Sanfilippo Syndrome: MPS III (see Complex Carbohydrate Metabolic Disorders)

Satoyoshi Syndrome [600705]

Clinical features:	Short stature, alopecia, diarrhoea and multiple skeletal abnormalities consequent upon recurrent injury due to violent muscle spasms.
Radiographic features:	Metaphyseal changes, epiphyseal slipping, cystic lesions in bone, acro-osteolysis, generalised osteolysis, fatigue fractures, precocious osteo-arthrosis.
Genetics:	Unknown.
Other considerations:	The majority of affected persons have been documented in Japan. The pathogenesis of the muscle spasms is unknown.
References:	Ehlayel MS, Lacassie Y (1995). Satoyoshi syndrome: an unusual postnatal multisystemic disorder. Am J Med Genet 57:620–625
	Ikegawa S, Nagano A, Satoyashi E (1993) Skeletal abnormalities in Satoyoshi's syndrome: a radiographic study of eight cases. Skeletal Radiol 22:321–324

Scapuloiliac Dysplasia (Pelvis-shoulder Dysplasia or Kosenow-Sinios Syndrome) [169550]

Clinical features:	Gross hypoplasia of the scapula, ilia and clavicles. Abnormalities of the eyes, ribs and lower spine may be present.
Radiographic features:	As above.
Genetics:	AD?
Other considerations:	Very rare.
References:	Kosenow W, Niederle J, Sinios A (1970). Becken-Schulter-Dysplasie. Fortschr Roentgenstr 113:39–48

Scheie Syndrome: MPS I-S (see Complex Carbohydrate Metabolic Disorders)

Schneckenbecken Dysplasia [269250]

Clinical features: Lethal neonatal short-limbed dwarfism.

Radiographic features: The iliac bones have medial protuberances that produce a pathognomonic "snail-like" appearance on pelvic radiographs; vertebrae are hypoplastic, ribs are short and clavicles are handlebar shaped. The limb bones are short with splayed ends.

Genetics: AR.

Other considerations: Rare.

References: Borochowitz Z, Jones KL, Silbey R, Adomian G, Lachman R, Rimoin DL (1986). A distinct lethal neonatal chondrodysplasia with snail-like pelvis: Schneckenbecken dysplasia. Am J Med Genet 25:47–59.

Camera G, Scarano G, Tronci A, La Cava G, Mastroiacovo P (1991). "Snail-like pelvis" chondrodysplasia: a further case report. Am J Med Genet 40:513–514

Schwartz Syndrome (see Myotonic Chondrodysplasia)

Sclerosteosis [269500]

Clinical features: Gigantism, prominent asymmetrical mandible. Variable syndactyly of the 2nd and 3rd fingers with radial deviation of the terminal phalanges and nail dysplasia. Compression of 7th and 8th cranial nerves.

Radiographic features: Generalised osteosclerosis with hyperostosis, predominantly of the skull. Hypotubulation of the tubular bones with marked undermodelling in the extremities.

Genetics: AR.

Other considerations: More than 60 affected persons in the Afrikaner population of South Africa, otherwise very rare.

References: Beighton P, Cremin B, Hamersma H (1976). The radiology of sclerosteosis. Br J Radiol 49:934–939

Beighton P (1988). Sclerosteosis. J Med Genet 25:200–203

Seckel Syndrome (Osteodysplastic, Primordial or Bird-headed Dwarfism) [210600; 210710; 210720]

Clinical features:	Small stature, mental deficiency, microcephaly, characteristic facies.
Radiographic features:	Hypoplasia of proximal ulna and proximal radius, dislocation of hips, 11 ribs.
Genetics:	AR, heterogeneous.
Other considerations:	The radiographic features are variable and non-diagnostic. Several forms of osteodysplastic primordial dwarfism with numerical designations have been proposed.
References:	Haan EA, Furness ME, Knowles S, Morris LL, Scott G, Svigos JM, Vigneswaren R (1989). Osteodysplastic primordial dwarfism: report of a further case with manifestations similar to those of types I and III. Am J Med Genet 33:224–227
	Hayani A, Suarez CR, Molnar Z, Le Beau M, Goodwin J (1994). Acute myeloid leukaemia in a patient with Seckel syndrome. J Med Genet 31:148–149
	Masuno M, Imaizumi K, Nishimura G, Kurosawa K, Makita Y, Shimazaki Y, Kuroki Y (1995). Osteodysplastic primordial dwarfism: a case with features of type II. Clin Dysmorph 4:57–62
	Shanske A, Caride DG, Menasse-Palmer L, Bogdanow A, Marion RW (1997). Central nervous system anomalies in Seckel syndrome: report of a new family and review of the literature. Am J Med Genet 70:155–158

SEMDJL (see Spondylo-epi-metaphyseal Dysplasia with Joint Laxity)

Shokeir Syndrome (Pena–Shokeir Syndrome; see Cerebro-oculo-facio-skeletal Syndrome)

Short Rib-Polydactyly Syndromes

Some doubt exists concerning the nosological status of the short rib syndromes. All forms present as lethal micromelic dwarfism with thoracic constriction and polydactyly. The relationship of the bony features to foetal maturity may be significant. Inheritance is AR in every instance.

Type I: Saldino–Noonan [263530]

Radiographic features: Narrow elongated thorax with short ribs. Distorted vertebral bodies with incomplete coronal clefts. Shortened sacro-iliac notches. Short tubular bones with triradiate ends. (fairly common).

References: Richardson MM, Beaudet AL, Wagner ML, Malini S, Rosenberg HS, Lucci JA Jr (1977). Prenatal diagnosis of recurrence of Saldino–Noonan dwarfism. J Pediatr 91:467–471
Saldino RM, Noonan CD (1972). Severe thoracic dystrophy with striking micromelia, abnormal osseous development, including the spine, and multiple visceral abnormalities. Am J Roentgenol 114:257–261

Type II: Majewski [263520]

Radiographic features: Narrow, elongated thorax with short ribs. Disproportionate shortening of the tibia. Normal pelvis and spine. (very rare).

Reference: Cooper CP, Hall CM (1982). Lethal short rib-polydactyly syndrome of the Majewski type: A report of three cases. Radiology 144(3):513–517
Neri G,, Gurrieri F, Genuardi M (1995). Oral-facial-skeletal syndromes. Am J Med Genet 59:365–368

Type III: Verma-Naumoff (Lethal Thoracic Dysplasia) [263510]

Radiographic features: Short ribs, marginal spur on femora. Abnormal ilia.

References: Naumoff P, Young LW, Mazer J, Amortegula AAJ (1977). Short rib-polydactyly syndrome type 3. Radiology 122:443–446
Wu M-H, Kuo P-L, Lin S-J (1995). Prenatal diagnosis of recurrence of short rib-polydactyly syndrome. Am J Med Genet 55:279–284

Type IV: Beemer-Langer [269860]

Radiographic features: Similar to type II, but the tibia is different. Polydactyly may be absent.

References: Beemer FA, Langer LO, Klep-de-Pater JM, Hemmes AM, Bylsma JB, Pauli RM, Myers TL, Haws CC (1983). A new short rib syndrome: report of two cases. Am J Med Genet 14:115–123

Hennekam RCM (1991). Short rib syndrome – Beemer type in sibs. Am J Med Genet 40:230–233

Lurie IW (1994). Further delineation of the Beemer-Langer syndrome using concordance rates in affected sibs. Am J Med Genet 50:313–317

Unclassifiable

A number of intermediate or unclassifiable forms of short rib polydactyly have been documented.

References: Martinez-Frias ML, Bermejo E, Urioste M, Egues J, Lopez Soler JA (1993). Short rib-polydactyly syndrome (SRPS) with anencephaly and other central nervous system anomalies. Am J Med Genet 47:782–287

Martinez-Frias ML, Bermejo E, Urioste M, Huertas H, Arroyo I (1993). Lethal short rib-polydactyly syndromes: further evidence for their overlapping in a continuous spectrum. J Med Genet 30:937–941

Sarafoglou K, Funai EF, Fefferman N, Zajac L, Geneiser N, Paidas MJ, Greco A, Wallerstein R (1999). Short rib-polydactyly syndrome: more evidence of a continuous spectrum. Clin Genet 56:145–148

Short Spine Dysplasia (see Brachyolmia)

Shwachman Syndrome (see Metaphyseal Chondrodysplasia and Bone Marrow Dysfunction)

Sialidoses (see Complex Carbohydrate Metabolic Disorders)

Silver Syndrome (see Russell–Silver Syndrome)

Singleton–Merten Syndrome [182250]

Clinical features: Generalised muscular weakness with secondary hip and foot deformities. Aortic stenosis. Psoriatic skin lesions. Dental dysplasia.

Radiographic features: Progressive calcification of the aorta beginning in childhood. Osteoporosis. Expanded medullary cavities of the metacarpals and metatarsals.

Genetics: AD.

Other considerations: Very rare.

Reference: Gay BB, Kuhn JP (1976). A syndrome of widened medullary cavities of bone, aortic calcification, abnormal dentition and muscular weakness (the Singleton–Merten syndrome). Radiology 118:389–394

Smith–Lemli–Opitz Syndrome [270400]

Clinical features: Small stature, failure to thrive, mental retardation. Peculiar facies. The diagnosis can be clinched by demonstration of faulty cholesterol synthesis.

Radiographic features: Inconsistent dislocation of the hips, punctate epiphyses during infancy, vertical talus.

Genetics: AR.

Other considerations: Probably fairly common but underdiagnosed.

References: Bialer MG, Penchaszadeh VB, Kahn E, Libes R, Krigsman G, Lesser ML (1987). Female external genitalia and mullerian duct derivatives in a 46,XY infant with the Smith–Lemli–Opitz syndrome. Am J Med Genet 28:723–731

Opitz JM, Penchaszadeh VB, Holt MC, Spano LM (1987). Smith–Lemli–Opitz (RSH) syndrome bibliography. Am J Med Genet 28:745–750

Seller MJ, Flinter FA, Docherty Z, Fagg N, Newbould M (1997). Phenotypic diversity in the Smith–Lemli–Opitz syndrome. Clin Dysmorph 6:69–73

Smith–McCort Syndrome (see Dyggve–Melchior–Clausen Dysplasia)

Sotos Syndrome (see Cerebral Gigantism)

Split-hand Split-foot Malformation (SHFM) [183600]

Clinical features:	Classically, the hands or feet are represented by two large digits or by monodactyly. Very variable in severity and extent.
Radiographic features:	Enlarged dysplastic digits.
Genetics:	AD with variable expression. Anomalous modes of transmission have been documented.
Other considerations:	The term "lobster claw malformation" is sometimes used for the SHFM. Ectrodactyly of this type may occur in combination with scalp defects in the Adams-Oliver syndrome [100300] and with facial clefts and ectodermal involvement (see EEC Syndrome [129900]). It is also a component of a few rare syndromes.
References:	Jarvik GP, Patton MA, Homfray T, Evans JP (1994). Non-Mendelian transmission in human developmental disorder: split hand/split foot. Am J Hum Genet 55:710–713
	Spranger M, Schapera J (1988). Anomalous inheritance in a kindred with split hand, split foot malformation. Europ J Pediatr 147:202–205
	Viljoen DL, Beighton P (1984). The split-hand and split-foot anomaly in a Central African Negro population. Am J Med Genet 19:545–552

Sponastrime Dysplasia [271510]

Clinical features:	Short-limbed dwarfism with depressed nasal bridge, frontal bossing and joint laxity. Mental retardation is a feature of a variant form.
Radiographic features:	Metaphyseal striations. Mild vertebral dysplasia in childhood.
Genetics:	AR.

Other considerations: The term "sponastrime" pertains to the spondy-
                           lar, nasal and metaphyseal manifestations.

References: Lachman RS, Stoss H, Spranger J (1989). SPO-
                           NASTRIME dysplasia: a radiologic-pathologic
                           correlation. Pediat Radiol 19:417–424
                           Langer LO Jr, Beals RK, LaFranchi S, Scott CL Jr,
                           Sockalosky JJ (1996). Sponastrime dysplasia:
                           five new cases and review of nine previously
                           published cases. Am J Med Genet 63:20–27
                           Verloes A, Misson J-P, Dubru J-M, Jamblin P, Le
                           Merrer M (1995). Heterogeneity of SPONAS-
                           TRIME dysplasia: delineation of a variant form
                           with severe mental retardation. Clin Dysmorph
                           4:208–215

Spondylocostal Dysostosis (Spondylothoracic Dysplasia) [122600; 277300]

Clinical features: Shortening of the trunk and neck, malformation
                          of the chest, scoliosis.

Radiographic features: Malsegmentation of the spine, hypoplastic or
                          dysplastic ribs.

Genetics: AD, mild. AR, severe (heterogeneous).

Other considerations: This group of disorders is rare but very hetero-
                          geneous. The spondylothoracic dysostoses belong
                          to the same general category.

References: Karnes PS, Day D, Berry SA, Pierpont MEM
                          (1991). Jarcho-Levin syndrome: four new cases
                          and classification of subtypes. Am J Med Genet
                          40:264–270
                          Kozlowski K (1981). Spondylo-costal dysplasia.
                          Severe and moderate types (report of 8 cases).
                          Australas Radiol 25:81–90
                          Mortier GR, Lachman RS, Bocian M, Rimoin DL
                          (1996). Multiple vertebral segmentation de-
                          fects: analysis of 26 new patients and review of
                          the literature. Am J Med Genet 61:310–319
                          Turnpenny PD, Thwaites RJ, Boulos FN (1991).
                          Evidence for variable gene expression in a large

inbred kindred with autosomal recessive spondylocostal dysostosis. J Med Genet 28:27–33

Spondylodysplasia (Platyspondylic Lethal Dysplasia) [151210]

Clinical features:
Lethal short-limbed neonatal dwarfism with a large head and very short limbs.

Radiographic features:
Marked platyspondyly, under-ossification of the cranial base, short thin ribs, hypoplasia of the pelvic bones, short wide tubular bones with metaphyseal cupping.

Genetics:
All reported cases have been sporadic and the mode of inheritance is unknown.

Other considerations:
Torrance, San Diego and Luton forms of spondylodysplasia have been proposed on a basis of histological changes in cartilage. These conditions have been regarded as variants of thanatophoric dysplasia [187600].

References:
Brodie SG, Kitoh H, Lachman RS, Nolasco LM, Mekikian PB, Wilcox WR (1999). Platyspondylic lethal skeletal dysplasia, San Diego Type, is caused by FGFR3 mutations. Am J Med Genet 84:476–480

Horton WA, Rimoin DL, Hollister DW, Lachman RS (1979). Further heterogeneity within lethal neonatal short-limbed dwarfism: The platyspondylic types. J Pediatr 94:736–742.

Jones KL, Jones KL, Miller K (1986). A new skeletal dysplasia syndrome with dwarfism, craniofacial anomalies, and unique radiographic findings. Am J Med Genet 23:751–757

Kaibara N, Yokoyama K, Nakano H (1983). Torrance type of lethal neonatal short-limbed platyspondylic dwarfism. Skeletal Radiol 10:17–19.

Kitoh H, Lachman RS, Brodie SG, Mekikian PB, Rimoin DL, Wilcox WR (1998). Extra pelvic ossification centres in thanatophoric dysplasia and platyspondylic lethal skeletal dysplasia-San Diego type. Pediatr Radiol 28:759–763

Spondyloenchondrodysplasia (Spondylometaphyseal Dysplasia with Enchondromatous Changes) [271550]

Clinical features: Stunted stature.

Radiographic features: Symmetrical, patchy, sclerotic and lucent areas in the metaphyses, platyspondyly, stubby digits.

Genetics: AR.

Other considerations: The condition is probably heterogeneous and there is considerable variation between affected families. Basal ganglia calcification may distinguish a specific form of spondyloenchondromatosis.

References: Schoor S, Legum C, Ochshorn M (1976). Spondyloenchondrodysplasia: enchondromatosis with severe platyspondyly in two brothers. Radiology 118:133–139

Menger H, Kruse K, Spranger J (1989). Spondyloenchondrodysplasia. J Med Genet 26:93–99

Zack P, Beighton P (1995). Spondyloenchondromatosis: syndromic identity and evolution of the phenotype. Am J Med Genet 55:478–482

Spondylo-epi-metaphyseal Dysplasia [271650; 601096; 120140]

Clinical features: Rhizomelic dwarfism with spinal malalignment.

Radiographic features: Irregularity of the epiphyses and metaphyses of the limb bones. Platyspondyly.

Genetics: AD and AR (heterogeneous).

Other considerations: The Irapa [271650], and Strudwick [184250] forms of SEMD are well recognised. There is considerable residual heterogeneity.

References: Hall MH, Elçioglu NH, Shaw DG (1998). A distinct form of spondyloepimetaphyseal dysplasia with multiple dislocations. J Med Genet 35:566–572

Hernandez A, Ramirez ML, Nazara Z, Ocampo R, Ibarra B, Cantu JM (1980). Autosomal recessive spondylo-epi-metaphyseal dysplasia (Irapa type) in a Mexican family: delineation of the syndrome. Am J Med Genet 5:179–188

Kozlowski K, Budzinska A (1966). Combined metaphyseal and epiphyseal dysostosis. Nouv Presse Med 5:319–324

Kozlowski K, Bieganski T, Gardner J, Beighton P (1999). Osteochondrodystrophies with marked platyspondyly and distinctive peripheral anomalies. Pediatr Radiol 29(1):1–5

Langer LO Jr, Wolfson BJ, Scott CI Jr, Reid CS, Schidlow DV, Millar EA, Borns PF, Lubicky JP, Carpenter BLM (1993). Further delineation of spondylo-meta-epiphyseal dysplasia, short limb-abnormal calcification type, with emphasis on diagnostic features. Am J Med Genet 45:488–500

Spondylo-epi-metaphyseal Dysplasia with Joint Laxity (SEMDJL) [271640]

Clinical features: Dwarfism, gross joint laxity, dislocations, progressive intractable spinal malalignment. Poor long-term prognosis.

Radiographic features: Moderate dysplastic changes throughout the spine, epiphyses and metaphyses of the long bones. Broad femoral necks with metaphyseal cysts and coxa valga deformity. Retarded bone age.

Genetics: AR.

Other considerations: More than 20 examples have been recognised, the majority in South Africa in families of Dutch-German stock.

References: Beighton P, Kozlowski K (1980). Spondylo-epi-metaphyseal dysplasia with joint laxity. Skeletal Radiol 5:205–212

Beighton P, Gericke G, Kozlowski K, Grobler L (1984). The manifestations and natural history of spondylo-epi-metaphyseal dysplasia with joint laxity. Clin Genet 26:308–317

Beighton P (1994). Spondyloepimetaphyseal dysplasia with joint laxity. (SEMDJL). J Med Genet 31:136–140

Spondylo-epiphyseal Dysplasia (SED)

In addition to the classical SED Congenita and Tarda forms (see below), many other types of SED have been proposed. The best recognised of these are the mild AD forms [120140] including Namaqualand Hip Dysplasia. The AR Toledo variety of SED [271630] is also well established although it is sometimes regarded as a variety of brachyolmia [271530]. SED is associated with the nephrotic syndrome in Schimke Immuno-osseous Dysplasia [242900]. Other forms of SED include the AR tarda type [271600], SED Stanescu type, and a form with antibody deficiency and retinal dystrophy. Mseleni joint disease in South Africa and Handigodu disease in India have the general manifestations of severe SED, as has progressive pseudo-rheumatoid arthropathy [208230].

References:

Agarwal SS, Phadke SR, Fredlund V, Viljoen DL, Beighton P (1997). Mseleni and Handigodu familial osteoarthropathies: syndromic identity? Am J Med Genet 72(4):435–439

Beighton P, Christy G, Learmonth ID (1984). Namaqualand hip dysplasia: an autosomal dominant entity. Am J Med Genet 19:161–169

Grain L, Duke O, Thompson G, Davies EG (1994). Toledo type brachyolmia. Arch Dis Child 71:448–449

Kohn G, Elrayyes ER, Makadmah I, Rosler A, Grunebaum M (1987). Spondyloepiphyseal dysplasia tarda: a new autosomal recessive variant with mental retardation. J Med Genet 24:366–377

Nishimura G, Saitoh Y, Okuzumi S, Imaizumi K, Hayasaka K, Hashimoto M (1998). Spondyloepiphyseal dysplasia with accumulation of glycoprotein in the chondrocytes: spondyloepiphyseal dysplasia, Stanescu type. Skeletal Radiol 27:188–194

Roifman CM (1999). Antibody deficiency, growth retardation, spondyloepiphyseal dysplasia and retinal dystrophy: a novel syndrome. Clin Genet 55:103–109

Santavá A, Zapletalová J, Michálková K, Hanáková S, Kopriva F, Santavy J, Dusek J, Kleinová D (1994). Spondyloepiphyseal dysplasia with nephrotic syndrome (Schimke immunoosseous dysplasia). Am J Med Genet 49:270–273

Saraiva JM, Dinis A, Resende C, Faria E, Gomes C, Correia AJ, Gil J, da Fonseca N (1999). Schimke immuno-osseous dysplasia: case report and review of 25 patients. J Med Genet 36:786–789

Viljoen D, Fredlund V, Ramesar R, Beighton P (1993). Brachydactylous dwarfs of Mseleni. Am J Med Genet 46:636–630

Spondylo-epiphyseal Dysplasia Congenita [183900]

Clinical features: Short trunk dwarfism, barrel chest, flat face, myopia. Relatively normal hands and feet.

Radiographic features: Anisospondyly, retarded bone age of the pelvis, coxa vara, normal extremities.

Genetics: AD.

Other considerations: Very heterogeneous. In mild forms, clinical problems may be virtually confined to the hip joints, with presentation as premature degenerative osteopathy. Mutations in the COL1A1 gene underlie this group of disorders.

References: Anderson IJ, Goldberg RB, Marion RW, Upholt WB, Tsipouras P (1990). Spondyloepiphyseal dysplasia congenita: genetic linkage to type II collagen (COL2A1). Am J Hum Genet 46:906–901

Kozlowski K, Masel J Morris L (1977). Dysplasia spondyloepiphysealis congenita – a critical analysis. Australas Radiol 21:260–280

Wynne-Davies R, Hall C (1982). Two clinical variants of spondylo-epiphyseal dysplasia congenita. J Bone Joint Surg [Br] 64(4):435–441

Spondylo-epiphyseal Dysplasia Tarda [313400]

Clinical features: Stunted stature with truncal shortening.

Radiographic features: Generalised moderate platyspondyly with a characteristic dorsal hump of the vertebral bodies. Small pelvis, dysplasia of femoral capital epiphyses, and early osteoarthritic changes.

Genetics: XL.

Other considerations:	The vertebral changes are pathognomonic in the classical form of SEDT. Although well recognised, this disorder is uncommon.
References:	Bannerman RM, Ingall GB, Mohn JF (1971). X-linked spondyloepiphyseal dysplasia tarda: clinical and linkage data. J Med Genet 8:291–301
	Bernard LE, Chitayat D, Weksberg R, Van Allen MI, Langlois S (1996). Linkage analysis of two Canadian families segregating for X linked spondyloepiphyseal dysplasia. J Med Genet 33:432–434
	Maroteaux P, Lamy M, Bernard J (1975). La dysplasie spondylo-épiphysare tardive. Presse Méd 65:1205–1208

Spondylo-epiphyseal Dysplasia with Diabetes Mellitus (Wolcott–Rallison Dysplasia) [226980]

Clinical features:	Dwarfism, early joint pain, renal failure, hepatosplenomegaly.
Radiographic features:	Mild platyspondyly, delayed ossification of fragmented epiphyses, resorption of femoral capital epiphyses.
Genetics:	AR.
Other considerations:	Rare.
References:	Al-Gazali LI, Makia S, Azzam A, Hall CM (1995). Wolcott–Rallison syndrome. Clin Dysmorph 4:227–233
	Stewart FJ, Carson DI, Thomas PS, Humphreys M, Thornton C, Nevin NC (1996). Wolcott–Rallison syndrome associated with congenital malformations and a mosaic deletion 15q11–12. Clin Genet 49:152–155
	Stoss H, Pewsch HJ, Pontz B, Otten A, Spranger J (1982). Wolcott–Rallison syndrome: diabetes mellitus and spondyloepiphyseal dysplasia. Eur J Pediatr 138:120–129.

Spondylometaphyseal Dysplasia (Kozlowski Type) [184252; 271600]

Clinical features:	Stature varies from normality to severe dwarfism. Minimal to marked shortening and malalignment of spine and limbs.
Radiographic features:	Variable, minimal to severe platyspondyly, minimal to severe metaphyseal changes, sometimes coxa vara.
Genetics:	AD, AR.
Other considerations:	Although rare, there is great heterogeneity in the SMD group of conditions.
References:	Kozlowski K, Prokop BE, Scougall JS, Silink M, Vines RH (1979). Spondylo-metaphyseal dysplasia. Fortschr Röntgenstr 130:222–230
	Kozlowski K, Cremin B, Beighton P (1980). Variability of spondylo-metaphyseal dysplasia, common type. Radiol Diagn 21:682–686
	Nores J-M, Dizien O, Remy J-M, Maroteaux P (1993). Two cases of spondylometaphyseal dysplasia: literature review and discussion of the genetic inheritance of the disease. J Rheum 20:170–172

Spondylometaphyseal Dysplasia, Other Forms

The Algerian [184253] Schmidt, Sutcliffe or "corner fracture" [184255], Goldblatt [184260] and XL types of SMD [313420] are well defined.

References:	Goldblatt J, Carman P, Sprague P (1991). Unique dwarfing, spondylometaphyseal skeletal dysplasia, with joint laxity and dentinogenesis imperfecta. Am J Med Genet39:170–172
	Langer, LO, Brill, PW, Ozonoff MB, Pauli RM, Wilson WG, Alford BA, Pavlov H, Drake DG (1990). Spondylometaphyseal dysplasia, corner fracture type: A heritable condition associated with coxa vara. Radiology 175:761–766
	Rybak M, Foley TP, Kozlowski K (1991). Spondylo-metaphyseal dysplasia Algerian type: confirmation of a new syndrome. Am J Med Genet 40:304–306

Spondylothoracic Dysplasia (see Spondylocostal Dysostosis)

Stanescu Syndrome (see Osteosclerosis)

Stickler Syndrome (see Arthro-ophthalmopathy)

Sturge-Weber Syndrome [185300]

Clinical features:	Unilateral "port wine" dermal lesion on the face in the distribution of the trigeminal nerve. Epilepsy.
Radiographic features:	"Double contour" calcification of the meninges.
Genetics:	Non-genetic?
Other considerations:	Common.
Reference:	Alonso A, Taboada D, Ceres L, Beltran J, Olague R, Nogues A (1979). Intracranial calcification in a neonate with the Sturge-Weber syndrome and additional problems. Pediatr Radiol 8:39–41
	Griffiths PD, Blaser S, Boodram MB, Armstrong D, Harwood-Nash D (1996). Choroid plexus size in young children with Sturge-Weber syndrome. Am J Neuroradiol 17:175–180
	Sujansky E, Conradi S (1995). Outcome of Sturge-Weber syndrome in 52 adults. Am J Med Genet 57:35–45

TAR Syndrome (see Radial Aplasia-Thrombocytopenia Syndrome)

Taybi–Linder Syndrome (Cephaloskeletal Dysplasia) [247400]

Clinical features:	Dwarfism with skeletal dysplasia and mental retardation. Lethal in infancy.
Radiographic features:	Microcephaly and vertebral coronal clefts.
Genetics:	AR.
Other considerations:	Very rare. This condition may be the same entity as osteodysplastic primordial dwarfism [210720].

References: Maroteaux P, Badoual J (1990). La chondrodys-
                       plasie microcephalique subletale: syndrome de
                       Taybi–Linder, nanisme microcephalique pri-
                       mordial de types I et III. Arch Franc Pediat
                       47:103–106
                       Taybi H, Linder D (1967). Congenital familial
                       dwarfism with cephaloskeletal dysplasia. Radi-
                       ology 89:275–281
                       Thomas PS, Nevin NC (1976). Congenital familial
                       dwarfism with cephalo-skeletal dysplasia (Tay-
                       bi–Linder syndrome). Ann Radiol (Paris)
                       19:187–192

Thanatophoric Dysplasia [187600; 187610]

Clinical features: Micromelic dwarfism with a large head and
                           normal trunk. Usually stillborn but occasional
                           survival into infancy has been reported.

Radiographic features: Generalised platyspondyly (H-shaped vertebral
                           bodies in AP projection), shortening and bowing
                           of the tubular bones, "telephone receiver" femora,
                           small sacro-iliac notches and narrowing of the
                           spinal canal. The lethal spondylodysplasias
                           [151210] have been termed thanatophoric dyspla-
                           sia variants.

Genetics: AD, new dominant mutation.

Other considerations: This condition is by far the most common of the
                           potentially lethal bone dysplasias of infancy.
                           Thanatophoric dysplasia type II, which is charac-
                           terised by straight femora and a cloverleaf skull, is
                           a less common variant.

References: Andersen PE Jr (1989). Prevalence of lethal
                               osteochondrodysplasias in Denmark. Am J
                               Med Genet 32:484–489
                           Connor JM, Connor RAC, Sweet EM, Gibson
                               AAM, Patrick WJA, McNay MB, Redford DHA
                               (1985). Lethal neonatal chondrodysplasias in
                               the West of Scotland, 1970–1983, with a
                               description of a thanatophoric dysplasia-like,
                               autosomal recessive disorder, Glasgow variant.
                               Am J Med Genet 22:243–253

Langer LO, Yang SS, Hall JG, Sommer A, Kottamasu S, Golabi R, Krassikoff N (1987). Thanatophoric dysplasia and cloverleaf skull. Am J Med Genet [Suppl] 3:167–179

Maroteaux P, Stanescu V, Stanescu R (1976). The lethal chondrodysplasias. Clin Orthop 114:31–35

Moir DH, Kozlowski K (1976). Long survival in thanatophoric dwarfism. Pediatr Radiol 5:123–125

Toxopachyostéose Diaphysaire Tibio-péronière (see Weismann–Netter–Stuhl Syndrome)

Treacher Collins Syndrome (Mandibulofacial Dysostosis) [154500]

Clinical features:	Mandibular and malar hypoplasia, microtia, deafness, antimongoloid slant to eyes, colobomata of lower eyelids.
Radiographic features:	Micrognathia.
Genetics:	AD with very variable clinical expression.
Other considerations:	The syndrome is relatively common. Apart from the cosmetic importance, it accounts for about 1% of all children with severe congenital deafness. The Nager form of acrofacial dysostosis [154400] is similar but has the additional feature of hypoplasia of the thumb and radius.
References:	Dixon MJ, (1996). Treacher Collins syndrome. Hum Molec Genet 1996:1391–1396 Hansen M, Lucarelli MJ, Whiteman DAH, Mulliken JB (1996). Treacher Collins syndrome: phenotypic variability in a family including an infant with arhinia and uveal colobomas. Am J Med Genet 61:71–74 McDonald MT, Gorski JL (1993). Nager acrofacial dysostosis. J Med Genet 30:779–782

Trichorhinophalangeal Dysplasia (Giedion–Langer Syndrome) [190350; 190351; 150230]

Clinical features:	Short stature, sparse, fine hair, pear-shaped nose, wide philtrum, swelling of the interphalangeal joints with axial deviation of the fingers.
Radiographic features:	Shortening of the tubular bones of the extremities, especially the distal phalanges of thumbs and toes, cone-shaped phalangeal epiphyses.
Genetics:	AD. Deletion in the long arm of chromosome 8 in some affected persons.
Other considerations:	Subcategorised into types I, II and III. Multiple exostoses are an additional feature of type II, while brachydactyly and the absence of exostoses and mental retardation characterise type III.
References:	Buhler EM, Buhler UK, Beutler C, Fessler R (1987). A final word on the tricho-rhino-phalangeal syndromes. Clin Genet 31:2730275 Giedion A (1998). Phalangeal cone-shaped epiphyses of the hand: their natural history, diagnostic sensitivity, and specificity in cartilage hair hypoplasia and the trichorhinophalangeal syndromes I and II. Pediatr Radiol 28:751–758 Kozlowski K, Harrington G, Barrylak A, Bartoszewica B (1977). Multiple exostoses – mental retardation syndrome, description of 2 childhood cases. Clin Pediatr 16:219–224 Nagai T, Nishimura G, Kasai H, Hasegawa T, Kato R, Ohashi H, Fukushima Y (1994). Another family with tricho-rhino-phalangeal syndrome type III (Sugio–Kajii syndrome). Am J Med Genet 49:278–280

Tuberous Sclerosis [191092]

Clinical features:	Facial adenoma sebaceum, periungual fibromata, variable mental retardation and epilepsy.
Radiographic features:	Irregular periosteal sclerosis, phalangeal cysts, peri-ventricular intracranial calcification.

Genetics: AD with variable expression. Genetically hetero-
                         geneous.

Other considerations: Tuberous sclerosis is common. The radiographic
                         manifestations are very variable and of little
                         diagnostic importance. Imaging studies of the
                         brain may be of value in detecting the condition
                         in asymptomatic persons.

References: Fryer AE, Chalmers AH, Osborne JP (1990). The
                         value of investigation for genetic counselling in
                         tuberous sclerosis. J Med Genet 27:217–223
                         Lustberg H, Gagliardi J, Lawson J (1999). Digital
                         enlargement in tuberous sclerosis. Skeletal
                         Radiol 28:116–118
                         Ruggieri M, Carbonara C, Magro G, Migone N,
                         Grasso S, Tine A, Pavone L, Gomez MR (1997).
                         Tuberous sclerosis complex: neonatal deaths in
                         three of four children of consanguineous, non-
                         expressing parents. J Med Genet 34:256–260
                         Winship IM, Connor JM, Beighton PH (1990).
                         Genetic heterogeneity in tuberous sclerosis:
                         phenotypic correlations. J Med Genet 27:418–
                         421

Tubular Stenosis (Kenny–Caffey Syndrome) [127000; 244460]

Clinical features: Short stature, transient hypoparathyroidism with
                         hypocalcaemia, anaemia.

Radiographic features: Narrowed medullary cavities with increased
                         cortical thickness, without widening of the
                         diaphyses, delayed cranial ossification.

Genetics: AD; AR.

Other considerations: The supposed AD form of the disorder may result
                         from a chromosomal microdeletion at 22q11. The
                         majority of reported examples of the AR form
                         have been in the Arab Bedouin community.

References: Franceschini P, Testa A, Bogetti G, Girardo E,
                         Guala A, Lopez-Bell O, Buzio G, Ferrario E,
                         Piccato E (1992): Kenny-Caffey syndrome in
                         two sibs born to consanguineous parents:
                         evidence for an autosomal recessive variant.
                         Am J Med Genet 42:112–116

Kozlowski K, Weisenbach J, Kosztolanyi G (1998). Kenny–Caffey syndrome. Case report. Radiol Med 95:669–671

Lee WK, Vargas A, Barnes J, Root AW (1983). The Kenny–Caffey syndrome: growth retardation and hypocalcemia in a young boy. Am J Med Genet 14(4):773–782

Sabry MA, Farag TI, Shaltout AA, Zaki M, Al-Mazidi Z, Abulhassan SJ, Al-Torki N, Quishawi A, Al Awadi SA (1999). Kenny–Caffey syndrome: an Arab variant? Clin Genet 55:44–49

Tumoral Calcinosis with Hyperphosphataemia [211900]

Clinical features: Painless masses usually near joints, in otherwise healthy children and young adults.

Radiographic features: Large localised calcified lesions in soft tissues overlying large joints.

Genetics: AR.

Other considerations: Very rare. Sometimes confused with fibrodysplasia ossificans progressiva but differs by virtue of circumscribed appearance and limited anatomical distribution.

References:
Clarke E, Swischuk LE, Hayden CK Jr (1984). Tumoral calcinosis, diaphysitis and hyperphosphatemia. Radiology 151:643–646

Metzker A, Eisentein B, Oren J, Samuel R (1988). Tumoral calcinosis revisited – common and uncommon features. Report of ten cases and review. Eur J Pediatr 147:128–132

Slavin RE, Wen J, Kumar D, Evans EB (1993). Familial tumoral calcinosis: a clinical, histopathologic, and ultrastructural study with an analysis of its calcifying process and pathogenesis. Am J Surg Path 17:788–802

Turner Syndrome

Clinical features: Females with absent secondary sexual characteristics due to ovarian dysgenesis. Short stature, webbed neck, broad chest, wide carrying angle, short 4th metacarpals, structural cardiac defects.

Radiographic features:	Short 4th metacarpals, variable skeletal abnormalities include flattening of the medial tibial condyles, retarded maturation and scoliosis.
Genetics:	XO chromosomal constitution, i.e. female with a missing X chromosome.
Other considerations:	The Turner syndrome occurs in about 1 in 3,000 females. Mosaics and other chromosomal variants that produce partial manifestations are fairly common.
References:	Cleveland RH, Done S, Correia JA, Crawford JD, Kushner DC, Herman TE (1985). Small carpal bone surface area, a characteristic of Turner's syndrome. Pediatr Radiol 15:168–172
	Rzymski K, Kosowicz J (1975). The skull in gonadal dysgenesis: a roentgenometric study. Clin Radiol 26:379–384

Van Buchem Disease (see Endosteal Hyperostosis, van Buchem Form)

VATER or VACTERL Association (see MURCS Association)

Verma-Naumoff Syndrome (see Short Rib Syndrome Type III)

Vitamin D-Resistant Rickets (Hypophosphataemia; see Rickets)

Von Recklinghausen Disease (see Neurofibromatosis)

Weaver Syndrome [277590]

Clinical features:	Prenatal onset of excessive size, peculiar facies, broad thumbs, thin deep-set nails.
Radiographic features:	Advanced bone age, broad distal metaphyses in the long bones, dysplastic vertebral bodies.
Genetics:	AR.
Other considerations:	Usually lethal in childhood. The nosological status of the Weaver syndrome is uncertain.
References:	Cole TRP, Dennis NR, Hughes HE (1992). Weaver syndrome. J Med Genet 29:332–337

Dumic M, Vukovic J, Cvitkovic M, Medica I
(1993). Twins and their mildly affected mother
with Weaver syndrome. Clin Genet 44:338–340
Teebi AS, Sundareshan TS, Hammouri MY, Al-
Awadi SA, Al-Saleh QA (1989). A new autosomal recessive disorder resembling Weaver
syndrome. Am J Med Genet 33:479–482

Weismann–Netter–Stuhl Syndrome (Toxopachyostéose Diaphysaire Tibio-péronière) [112350]

Clinical features: Anterior curvature of the shins with mental deficiency and variable short stature.

Radiographic features: Bowing of the tibia and fibula with diaphyseal cortical endosteal hyperostosis. Kyphoscoliosis, iliac squaring and calcification of the falx cerebri are variable.

Genetics: AD?

Other considerations: There is some doubt concerning the independent syndromic identity of this disorder.

References: Amendola MA, Brower AC, Tisnado J (1980). Weismann–Netter–Stuhl syndrome: toxopa-chyostéose diaphysaire tibio-péronière. Am J Roentgen 135:1211–1215
Robinow M, Johnson GF (1988). The Weismann–Netter syndrome. Am J Med Genet 29:573–579

Weissenbacher–Zweymüller Syndrome (Micrognathic Dwarfism) [277610]

Clinical features: Neonatal micromelic dwarfism with micrognathia and cleft palate.

Radiographic features: Marked metaphyseal widening, cleft vertebrae, platyspondyly, delayed development of femoral capital epiphyses.

Genetics: AR.

Other considerations: Rare. In survivors the radiographic configuration of the long bones reverts towards normality. An aetiological relationship with the Stickler syndrome has been proposed.

References:

Chemke J, Carmi R, Galil A, Bar-Ziv Y, Ben-Ytzhak I, Zurkowski L (1992).Weissenbacher–Zweymüller syndrome: a distinct autosomal recessive skeletal dysplasia. Am J Med Genet 43:989–995

Kelly TE, Wells HH, Tuck, KB (1982). The Weissenbacher–Zweymüller syndrome: possible neonatal expression of the Stickler syndrome. Am J Med Genet 11(1):113–119

Ramer JC, Eggli K, Rogan PK, Ladda RL (1993). Identical twins with Weissenbacher–Zweymüller syndrome and neural tube defect. Am J Med Genet 45:614–618

Werner Syndrome [277700]

Clinical features: Sclerosis of the skin, cataracts, premature ageing of the face and blood vessels, stunted stature.

Radiographic features: Subcutaneous calcification.

Genetics: AR.

Other considerations: Malignancy is frequent in affected persons. The majority of reports of affected persons have emanated from Japan. The Werner type of mesomelic dysplasia is a different entity.

References:

Epstein CJ, Martin GM, Schultz AL, Motulsky AG (1966). Werner's syndrome: a review of its symptomatology, natural history, pathologic features, genetics and relationship to the natural ageing process. Medicine 45:177–222

Goto M, Tanimoto K, Horiuchi Y, Sasazuki T (1981). Family analysis of Werner's syndrome: a survey of 42 Japanese families with a review of the literature. Clin Genet 19:8–15

Yu E-E, Oshima J, Wijsman E, Nakura J, Miki T, Piussan C, Matthews S, Fu Y-H, Mulligan J, Martin GM, Schellenberg GD (1997). Werner's Syndrome Collaborative Group: Mutations in the consensus helicase domains of the Werner syndrome gene. Am J Hum Genet 60:330–341

Whistling Face Syndrome (see Freeman–Sheldon Syndrome)

Wildervanck Syndrome (see Cervico-oculo-acoustic Syndrome)

Wolcott–Rallison Dysplasia (see Spondylo-epiphyseal Dysplasia with Diabetes Mellitus)

Worth Syndrome (see Endosteal Hyperostosis, Worth Type)

Zellweger Syndrome (see Cerebro-hepato-renal Syndrome)

Appendix A

Textbooks and Monographs

Beighton P (1993) McKusick's heritable disorders of connective tissue, 5th edn. CV Mosby, St Louis, MO

Beighton P (1988) Inherited disorders of the skeleton, 2nd edn. Churchill Livingstone, Edinburgh

Beighton P, Cremin BJ (1980) Sclerosing bone dysplasias. Springer, Berlin

Beighton P, Grahame R, Bird H (1999) Hypermobility of joints, 3rd edn. Springer, Berlin

Buyse ML (ed) (1990) Birth defects encyclopaedia. Blackwell Scientific, Cambridge, MA

Connor JM (1983) Soft tissue ossification. Springer, Berlin

Cremin BJ, Beighton P (1978) Bone dysplasias in infancy. A radiological atlas. Springer, Berlin

Donnai D, Winter RM (1995) Congenital malformation syndromes. Chapman & Hall, London

Gorlin RJ, Cohen MM, Levin LS (1990) Syndromes of the head and neck, 3rd edn. McGraw-Hill, New York

Horan F, Beighton P (1982) Orthopaedic problems in inherited skeletal disorders. Springer, Berlin

Jones KL (1997) Smith's recognisable patterns of human malformation, 5th edn. WB Saunders, Philadelphia, PA

Kaufman JH (ed) (1973) Intrinsic diseases of bone. Progress in Pediatric Radiology, vol 4. Karger, Basel

Maroteaux P (1979) Bone diseases of children. Lippincott, Philadelphia, PA

McKusick VA (1998) Mendelian inheritance in man, 12th edn. Johns Hopkins Press, Baltimore, MA

Mueller RF, Young ID (1998) Emery's elements of medical genetics. Harcourt Brace, London

Papadatos CJ, Bartsocas CS (eds) (1982) Skeletal dysplasias. Progress in clinical and biological research, vol 104. Alan R Liss, New York

Poznanski AK (1974) The hand in radiologic diagnosis. WB Saunders, Philadelphia, PA

Royce PM, Steinmann B (1993) Connective tissue and its heritable disorders. Wiley-Liss, New York

Spranger JW, Langer LO, Wiedemann HR (1974) Bone dysplasias. An atlas of constitutional disorders of skeletal development. WB Saunders, Philadelphia, PA

Stanbury JB, Wyngaarden JB, Fredrickson DS, Goldstein JL, Brown MS (1983) The metabolic basis of inherited diseases, 5th edn. McGraw-Hill, New York

Taybi H (1990) Radiology of syndromes, 3rd edn. Year Book Medical Publishers, Chicago, IL

Temtamy SA, McKusick VA (1978) The genetics of hand malformations. Birth Defects: Original Article Series, XIV (3)

Warkany J (1971) Congenital malformations. Year Book Medical Publishers, Chicago, IL

Wiedemann HR, Grosse KR, Dibbern H (1988) An atlas of characteristic syndromes. Wolfe, Stuttgart

Wynne-Davies R, Hall CM, Apley AG (1985) Atlas of skeletal dysplasias. Churchill Livingstone, Edinburgh

Appendix B

International Nomenclature and Classification of the Osteochondrodysplasias (1997)

International Working Group on Constitutional Diseases of Bone

Pediatr Radiol (1998) 28: 737–744*

Preamble

The International Working Group on Bone Dysplasias met in Los Angeles, California on August 5 and 6, 1997, to perform the third official revision of the 1972 Paris Nomenclature of Constitutional Disorders of Bone. In the last revision (1992), the classification was reoriented on radiodiagnostic and morphologic criteria and grouped morphologically similar disorders into "families" of disorders based on presumed pathogenetic similarities.

In the present, newly revised nomenclature, the families of disorders were to some extent rearranged based on recent etiopathogenetic information concerning the gene and/or protein defect in these disorders. In those disorders in which the basic defect was well documented, they were regrouped into distinct families, in which the component disorders were due to mutations in the same gene. These included the "achondroplasia group" of disorders with mutations in fibroblast growth factor receptor 3; the "diastrophic dysplasia" group of disorders, with mutations in the dia-

*Reproduced by permission of Professor Ralph S. Lachman, and Springer-Verlag

David L. Rimoin, MD, Ph.D. (Los Angeles) (Chair); Clair A. Francomano, MD (Bethesda); Andres Giedion, MD (Zurich); Christine Hall, MD (London); Ilkka Kaitila, MD (Helsinki); Dan Cohn, Ph.D. (Los Angeles); Robert Gorlin, DDS (Minneapolis); Judith Hall, MD (Vancouver); William Horton, MD (Portland); Deborah Krakow, MD (Los Angeles); Martine Le Merrer, MD (Paris); Ralph Lachman, MD (Los Angeles); Stefan Mundlos, MD (Mainz); Andrew K. Posnanski, MD (Chicago); David Sillence, MD (Sydney); Jürgen Spranger, MD (Mainz); Matthew Warman, MD (Cleveland); Andrea Superti-Furga, MD (Zurich); and William Wilcox, MD (Los Angeles)

strophic dysplasia sulfate transporter gene; the "type II collagenopathies," with mutations in type II collagen; and the "type XI collagenopathies" with mutations in cartilage-oligomeric matrix protein (COMP). Several new groups of disorders were added, including the "lethal skeletal dysplasia" group with fragmented bones and the "miscellaneous neonatal severe dysplasia" group. Other families were renamed, such as the "osteodysplastic slender bone group". Because of the large number of dysplasias with increased bone density, this group was subdivided into three new families: "increased bone density without modi-fication of bone shape"; "increased bone density with diaphyseal involvement", and "increased bone density with metaphyseal involvement".

References for most of the skeletal dysplasias can be obtained through a text such as the third chapter of the Taybi/Lachman book The Radiology of Syndromes, Metabolic Disorders and Skeletal Dysplasias, 4th Edition, or through on-line access of the Mendelian Inheritance in Man (OMIM) on the Internet directly or by accessing the International Skeletal Dysplasia Web Site (http://www.csmc.edu/genetics/skeledys/) where each disorder is hyperlinked to OMIM.

The authors have attempted to estimate the relative frequency of these conditions in terms of their own experience and a review of the literature:

**** : 1000+ cases
*** : 100–1000 cases
** : 20–100 cases
* : Less than 20 cases

In the updated 1997 International Classification, some conditions have been sub-categorised by virtue of genetic heterogeneity. It has not always been possible to estimate the relative frequencies of the individual members of these sub-groups.

Abbreviations: AD = Autosomal dominant; AR = Autosomal recessive; XLD = X-linked dominant; XLR = X-linked recessive; Sp = Sporadic; OMIM = Mendelian Inheritance in Man (McKusick's catalogue online)

International Classification of Osteochondrodysplasias

Osteochondrodysplasias	Inheritance	OMIM	Present at birth	Frequency
1. Achondroplasia group				
Thanatophoric dysplasia, type I	AD	187600	+	***
Thanatophoric dysplasia, type II	AD	187610	+	**
Achondroplasia	AD	100800	+	****
Hypochondroplasia	AD	146000	–	***
Other FGFR3 disorders				
2. Spondylodysplastic and other perinatally lethal groups				
Lethal platyspondylic skeletal dysplasias				
(San Diego type, Torrance type, Luton type)		270230	+	**
	SP	151210	+	
Achondrogenesis type 1A	AR	200600	+	**
3. Metatropic dysplasia group				
Fibrochondrogenesis	AR	228520	+	*
Schneckenbecken dysplasia	AR	269250	+	*
Metatropic dysplasia (various forms)	AD	156520	+	**
4. Short-rib dysplasia (SRP) (with or without polydactyly) group				
SRP type I, Saldino–Noonan	AR	263530	+	**
SRP type II, Majewski	AR	263520	+	*
SRP type III, Verma–Naumoff	AR	263510	+	*
SRP type IV, Beemer–Langer	AR	269860	+	*
Asphyxiating thoracic dysplasia (Jeune)	AR	208500	+	**
Chondroectodermal dysplasia (Ellis–van Creveld dysplasia)	AR	225500	+	***
5. Atelosteogenesis-omodysplasia group				
Atelosteogenesis type I (includes "boomerang dysplasia")	SP	108720	+	*
Omodysplasia I (Maroteaux)	AD	164745	+	*
Omodysplasia II (Borochowitz)	AR	258315	+	*
Otopalatodigital syndrome type II	XLR	304120	+	*
Atelosteogenesis type III	SP	108721	+	*
de la Chapelle dysplasia	AR	256050	+	*
6. Diastrophic dysplasia group				
Diastrophic dysplasia	AR	222600	+	***
Achondrogenesis 1B	AR	600972	+	*
Atelosteogenesis type II	AR	256050	+	*

Osteochondrodysplasias	Inheritance	OMIM	Present at birth	Frequency
7. Dyssegmental dysplasia group				
Dyssegmental dysplasia (Silverman–Handmaker type)	AR	224410	+	*
Dyssegmental dysplasia (Rolland–Desbuquois type)	AR	224400	+	*
8. Type II collagenopathies				
Achondrogenesis II (Langer–Saldino)	AD	200610	+	**
Hypochondrogenesis	AD	200610	+	*
Kniest dysplasia	AD	156550	+	**
Spondyloepiphyseal dysplasia (SED) congenita	AD	183900	+	**
Spondyloepimetaphyseal dysplasia (SEMD) Strudwick type	AD	184250	+	*
SED with brachydactyly	AD			*
Mild SED with premature onset arthrosis	AD		–	**
Stickler dysplasia (heterogeneous, some not linked to COL2A1)	AD	108300	+	**
9. Type XI collagenopathies				
Stickler dysplasia (heterogeneous)	AD	184840	+	**
Osteospondylomegaepiphyseal dysplasia (OSMED)	AR	215150	+	*
10. Other spondyloepi(meta)physeal [SE(M)D] dysplasias				
X-linked spondyloepiphyseal dysplasia tarda	XLD	313400	–	**
Other late-onset spondyloepi(meta)physeal dysplasias (Irapa) (Namaqualand)	AR	271650	–	***
Progressive pseudorheumatoid dysplasia	AR	208230	–	**
Dyggve–Melchior–Clausen dysplasia	AR	223800	+	**
Wolcott–Rallison dysplasia	AR	226980	–	*
Immuno-osseous dysplasia–Schimke	AR	242900	+	*
Opsismodysplasia	AR	258480	+	*
Chondrodystrophic myotonia	AR	258480	+	**
(Schwartz Jampel), type 1, type 2	AR	255800	+	**
Spondyloepiphyseal dysplasia with joint laxity	AR	271640	+	**
Sponastrime dysplasia	AR	271510	–	*
SEMD short limb-abnormal calcification type	AR	271665	+	*

Osteochondrodysplasias	Inheritance	OMIM	Present at birth	Frequency
11. Multiple epiphyseal dysplasias and pseudoachondroplasia				
Pseudoachondroplasia	AD	177170	–	***
Multiple epiphyseal dysplasia (MED)	AD	132400	–	***
(Fairbanks and Ribbing types)	AD	600204	–	?
Other MEDs	?	600969	–	?
12. Chondrodysplasia punctata (stippled epiphyses group)				
Rhizomelic type	AR	215100	+	**
Zellweger syndrome	AR	214100	+	**
Conradi–Hünermann type	XLD	302950	+	***
X-linked recessive type	XLR	302940	+	*
Brachytelephalangic type	XLR	302940	+	*
Tibial-metacarpal type	AD	118651	+	*
Vitamin K-dependent coagulation defect	AR	277450	+	*
Other acquired and genetic disorders including Warfarin embryopathy				
13. Metaphyseal dysplasias				
Jansen type	AD	156400	+	*
Schmid type	AD	156500	–	**
McKusick type (cartilage-hair hypoplasia	AR	250250	+	**
Metaphyseal anadysplasia	XLR?	309645	–	*
Metaphyseal dysplasia with pancreatic insufficiency and cyclic neutropenia. (Schwachman Diamond)	AR	260400	–	**
Adenosine deaminase deficiency	AD	102700	–	**
Metaphyseal chondrodysplasia-Spahr type	AR	250400	–	*
Acroscyphodysplasia (various types)	AR	250215	–	*
14. Spondylometaphyseal dysplasias (SMD)				
Spondylometaphyseal dysplasia (Kozlowski type)	AD	184252	+	**
Spondylometaphyseal dysplasia (Sutcliffe type)	AD	184255	+	**
SMD with severe genu valgum (includes Schmidt and Algerian types)	AD	184253	+	*
SMD Sedaghatian type	AR		+	*
Mild SMD different types			–	

Osteochondrodysplasias	Inheritance	OMIM	Present at birth	Frequency
15. Brachyolmia spondylodysplasias				
Hobaek (includes Toledo type)	AR	271530-630	–	*
Maroteaux type	AR		–	*
Autosomal dominant type	AD	113500	–	*
16. Mesomelic dysplasias				
Dyschondrosteosis (Leri-Weill)	AD	127300	–	**
Langer type (homozygous dyschondrosteosis)	AR	249700	+	*
Nievergelt type	AD	163400	+	*
Kozlowski-Reardon type	AR		+	*
Reinhardt-Pfeiffer type	AD	191400	+	*
Werner type	AD		+	*
Robinow type, dominant	AD	180700	–	*
Robinow type, recessive	AR	268310	–	*
Mesomelic dysplasia with synostosis	AD	600383	+	*
17. Acromelic and acromesomelic dysplasias				
Acromicric dysplasia	AD	102370	+	*
Geleophysic dysplasia	AR	231050	+	*
Weill-Marchesani dysplasia	AR	277600	+	*
Cranioectodermal dysplasia	AR	218330	+	*
Trichorhinophalangeal dysplasia type I	AD	190350	+	**
Trichorhinophalangeal dysplasia type II (Langer-Giedion)	AD	150230	+	**
Trichorhinophalangeal dysplasia, type III	AD	190351	+	?
Grebe dysplasia	AR	200700	+	**
Hunter-Thompson dysplasia	AR	201250	+	*
Brachydactyly type A1-A4	AD	112500-800	+	?
Brachydactyly type B	AD	113000	+	?
Brachydactyly type C	AD	133100	+	?
Brachydactyly type D	AD	113200	+	?
Brachydactyly type E	AD	113000	–	?
Pseudohypoparathyroidism (Albright hereditary osteodystrophy) various types			–	**
Acrodysostosis	SP(AD)	101800	–	**
Saldino–Mainzer dysplasia	AR	266920	–	*
Brachydactyly-hypertension dysplasia (Bilginturan)	AD	112410	+	*

Osteochondrodysplasias	Inheritance	OMIM	Present at birth	Frequency
Craniofacial conodysplasia	AD		+	*
Angel-shaped phalango-epiphyseal dysplasia (ASPED)	AD	105835	+	*
Acromesomelic dysplasia	AR	201250	+	**
Other acromesomelic dysplasias				
18. Dysplasias with prominent membranous bone involvement				
Cleidocranial dysplasia	AD	119600	+	***
Osteodysplasty, Melnick–Needles	XLD	309350	–	**
Precocious osteodysplasty (ter Haar dysplasia)	AR		+	*
Yunis–Varon dysplasia	AR	216340	+	*
19. Bent-bone dysplasia group				
Campomelic dysplasia	AD	114290	+	**
Kyphomelic dysplasia	?AR	211350	+	*
Stüve–Wiedemann dysplasia	AR	601559	+	*
20. Multiple dislocations with dysplasias				
Larsen syndrome	AD	150250	+	**
Larsen-like syndromes (including La Réunion Island type)	AR	245600	+	*
Desbuquois dysplasia	AR	251450	+	*
Pseudodiastrophic dysplasia	AR	264180	+	*
21. Dysostosis multiplex group				
Mucopolysaccharidosis IH	AR	252800	–	***
Mucopolysaccharidosis IS	AR	252800	–	**
Mucopolysaccharidosis II	XLR	309900	–	***
Mucopolysaccharidosis IIIA	AR	252900	–	***
Mucopolysaccharidosis IIIB	AR	252920	–	***
Mucopolysaccharidosis IIIC	AR	252930	–	***
Mucopolysaccharidosis IIID	AR	252940	–	***
Mucopolysaccharidosis IVA	AR	230500	–	**
Mucopolysaccharidosis IVB	AR	253010	–	**
Mucopolysaccharidosis VI	AR	253200	–	**
Mucopolysaccharidosis VII	AR	253200	–	**
Fucosidosis	AR	230000	–	**
α-Mannosidosis	AR	248500	–	**
β-Mannosidosis	AR	248510	–	**
Aspartylglucosaminuria	AR	208400	–	**
GM1 Gangliosidosis, several forms	AR	230500	+	**
Sialidosis, several forms	AR	256550	+/–	**
Sialic acid storage disease	AR	269920	+/–	**
Galactosialidosis, several forms	AR	256540		**

Osteochondrodysplasias	Inheritance	OMIM	Present at birth	Frequency
Multiple sulfatase deficiency	AR	272200	+/-	**
Mucolipidosis II	AR	252500	+	**
Mucolipidosis III	AR	252600	–	**

22. Osteodysplastic slender bone group

Type I osteodysplastic dysplasia	AR	210710	+	**
Type II osteodysplastic dysplasia	AR	210720	+	**
Microcephalic osteodysplastic dys.	AR		+	?

23. Dysplasias with decreased bone density

Osteogenesis imperfecta I (without opalescent teeth	AD	166200	+/-	
Osteogenesis imperfecta I (with opalescent teeth	AD	166240	+/-	
	AD	166240	+/-	
Osteogenesis imperfecta II	AD	166210	+	
	AR	259400	+	***
Osteogenesis imperfecta III	AD	259420	+	**
	AR	259420	+	
Osteogenesis imperfecta IV (without opalescent teeth)	AD	166220	+	***
Osteogenesis imperfecta IV (with opalescent teeth)	AD	166220	+	
Cole–Carpenter dysplasia	SP	112240	+	*
Bruck dysplasia	AR	259450	+	*
Singleton–Merten dysplasia	AD?	182250	**	
Osteopenia with radiolucent lesions of the mandible	AD	166260	*	
Osteoporosis-pseudoglioma dysplasia	AR	259770	–	**
Geroderma osteodysplasticum	AR	231070	–	**
Hyper IGE syndrome with osteopenia	AR	147060	–	*
Idiopathic juvenile osteoporosis	SP	259750	–	**

24. Dysplasias with defective mineralization

Hypophosphatasia-perinatal lethal and infantile forms	AR	241500	+	**
Hypophosphatasia adult form	AD	146300	–	**
Hypophosphataemic rickets	XLD	307800	–	***
Neonatal hyperparathyroidism	AR	239200	+	*
Transient neonatal hyperparathyroidism	AD	145980	+	*
with hypocalciuric hypercalcemia	AD	+		

Osteochondrodysplasias	Inheritance	OMIM	Present at birth	Frequency
25. Increased bone density without modification of bone shape				
Osteopetrosis				
Precocious type	AR	259700	+	**
Delayed type	AD	166600	–	**
Intermediate type	AR	259710	+	*
with renal tubular acidosis	AR	259730	+	**
Axial osteosclerosis				
Osteomesopyknosis	AD	166450	–	*
with bamboo hair	AR	266500	–	*
Pyknodysostosis	AR	265800	+	**
Osteosclerosis Stanescu type	AD	122900	+	*
Osteopathia striata				
Isolated	SP		–	?
with cranial sclerosis	AD	166500	–	**
Sponastrime dysplasia	AR	271510	+	*
Melorheostosis	SP	155950	–	**
Osteopoikilosis	AD	166700	–	**
Mixed sclerosing bone dysplasia	SP	–		
26. Increased bone density with diaphyseal involvement				
Diaphyseal dysplasia Camurati–Engelmann	AD	131300	–	**
Craniodiaphyseal dysplasia	?AR	218300	+	*
Lenz–Majewski dysplasia	SP	151050	+	*
Endosteal hyperostosis				
van Buchem type	AR	239100	–	**
Worth type	AD	144750	–	*
Sclerosteosis	AR	269500	–	**
with cerebellar hypoplasia	AR	213002	+	*
Kenny–Caffey dysplasia	AD,AR	127000	–	*
		244460	–	
Osteoectasia with hyperphosphatasia (Juvenile Pagets disease)	AR	239000	–	**
Diaphyseal dysplasia with anaemia	AR	231095	–	*
Diaphyseal medullary stenosis with bone malignancy (Hardcastle)	AD	112250	–	*

Osteochondrodysplasias	Inheritance	OMIM	Present at birth	Frequency
27. Increased bone density with metaphyseal involvement				
Pyle dysplasia	AR	265900	–	**
Craniometaphyseal dysplasia				
severe type	AR	218400	+	*
mild type	AD	123000	–	**
other types				
Frontometaphyseal dysplasia	XLR	305620	–	*
Dysosteosclerosis	AR	224300	–	*
	XLR			
Oculodentoosseous dysplasia	AD	164200	+	**
	AR	257850	+	*
Trichodentoosseous dysplasia	AD	190320	–	*
28. Neonatal severe osteosclerotic dysplasias				
Blomstrand dysplasia	AR	215045	+	*
Raine dysplasia	?	259775	+	*
Prenatal onset Caffey disease	?AR	114000	+	*
29. Lethal chondrodysplasias with fragmented bones				
Greenberg dysplasia	AR	215140	+	*
Dappled diaphyseal dysplasia	AR		+	*
Astley–Kendall dysplasia	AR		+	*
30. Disorganised development of cartilaginous and fibrous components of the skeleton				
Dysplasia ephysealis hemimelica	SP	127800	–	**
Multiple cartilaginous exostoses	AD	133700	–	***
	AD	133701	–	
	AD	600209	–	
Enchondromatosis, Ollier	SP	166000	–	**
Enchondromatosis with haemangiomata, (Maffucci)	SP	166000	–	**
Spondyloenchondromatosis	AR	271550	–	*
Spondyloenchondromatosis with basal ganglia calcification	AR		–	*
Dysspondyloenchondromatosis			–	*
Metachondromatosis	AD	156250		*
Osteoglophonic dysplasia	AD	166250	+	*
Genochondromatosis	AD	166000	–	*
Carpotarsal osteochondromatosis	AD	127820	–	*
Fibrous dysplasia (McCune–Allbright and others)	SP mosaic	174800	–	***
Jaffe–Campanacci	SP			
Fibrodysplasia ossificans progressiva	AD	135100	+	**
Cherubism	AD	118400	–	**
Cherubism with gingival fibromatosis	AR	135300	–	**

Osteochondrodysplasias	Inheritance	OMIM	Present at birth	Frequency
31. Osteolyses				
Multicentric carpal-tarsal osteolysis with and without nephropathy	AD	166300	–	**
Francois syndrome	AR	221800	–	*
Winchester syndrome	AR	277950	–	*
Torg syndrome	AR	259600	–	**
Hajdu–Cheney syndrome	AD	102500	–	*
Giacci familial neurogenic acroosteolysis	AR	201300	–	*
Mandibulo acral syndrome	AR	248370	–	*
Familial expansile osteolysis	AD	174810	–	**
Juvenile hyaline fibromatosis	AR	228600	+	*
32. Patella dysplasias				
Nail patella dysplasia	AD	161200	–	***
Scypho-patellar dysplasia	AD		+	*

Subject Index